Integrated
Patient Care
for the
Imaging
Professional

D1542408

Integrated Patient Care
for the
Imaging Professional

NINA KOWALCZYK, MS, RT(R)

Associate Technical Director of Radiology
The Ohio State University Hospitals
Adjunct Faculty, Radiography Program
The Ohio State University
Columbus, Ohio

KATHLEEN DONNETT, RN, RT(R)(CV)

Staff Nurse, Radiology Department
Riverside Methodist Hospital
Columbus, Ohio

with 204 illustrations

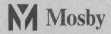 Mosby

St. Louis Baltimore Boston Carlsbad Chicago Naples New York Philadelphia Portland
London Madrid Mexico City Singapore Sydney Tokyo Toronto Wiesbaden

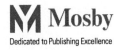

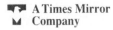

EDITOR: JEANNE ROWLAND
DEVELOPMENTAL EDITORIAL SERVICES: TOM LOCHHAAS
PROJECT MANAGER: LINDA MCKINLEY
PRODUCTION EDITOR: CATHERINE BRICKER
DESIGNER: ELIZABETH FETT
MANUFACTURING SUPERVISOR: THERESA FUCHS
COVER DESIGNER: GW GRAPHICS

Copyright © 1996 by Mosby-Year Book, Inc.

All rights reserved. No part of this publication may be reproduced, stored in a retrieval system, or transmitted, in any form or by any means, electronic, mechanical, photocopying, recording, or otherwise, without prior written permission from the publisher.

Permission to photocopy or reproduce solely for internal or personal use is permitted for libraries or other users registered with the Copyright Clearance Center, provided that the base fee of $4.00 per chapter plus $.10 per page is paid directly to the Copyright Clearance Center, 27 Congress Street, Salem, MA 01970. This consent does not extend to other kinds of copying, such as copying for general distribution, for advertising or promotional purposes, for creating new collected works, or for resale.

Printed in the United States of America

Composition by Graphic World, Inc.
Printing/binding by Rand McNally Book Services

Mosby-Year Book, Inc.
11830 Westline Industrial Drive
St. Louis, Missouri 63146

Library of Congress Cataloging-in-Publication Data

Kowalczyk, Nina.
   Integrated patient care for the imaging professional / by Nina
Kowalczyk, Kathleen Donnett.
       p.   cm.
   Includes bibliographical references and index.
   ISBN 0-8151-2545-3
   1. Radiography, Medical.   2. Radiologic technologists.   3. Medical
care.   4. Medical personnel and patient.   I. Donnett, Kathleen.
II. Title.
   [DNLM: 1. Diagnostic Imaging.   2. Radiology.   3. Professional-
Patient Relations.   WN 180 K88i 1996]
   RC78.K75   1996
   616.07'54—dc20
   DNLM / DLC
   for Library of Congress   95-49882
                                                            CIP

96 97 98 99 00 / 9 8 7 6 5 4 3 2 1

616.075
Kow

32.26

Dedication

ALTHOUGH I HAVE PRACTICED IN MANY AREAS OF THE RADIO-
logic technologic profession, the importance of the humanistic side
of our profession to patients and family members only recently had
a real-life impact on me. I dedicate this text to my father who passed
away during the writing of this patient-care textbook.

My father taught me many things during his lifetime, so it is only
appropriate that the last year of his life paralleled the writing of this
text. My father was a very caring and loving person who suffered
from both Parkinson's and Alzheimer's disease. Throughout his
battle with disease, his health and mental status progressively declined. He was unable to verbally communicate for the last few
months of his life but was still able to instill in me the importance
of the humanistic aspect of patient care. In a profession which is dri-
ven by technologic advances, it is easy to forget that each patient is
someone's loved one—a mother, a father, a child. Always remember
that each person you encounter deserves to be treated with dignity
and respect.

NK

As a senior in high school, when many of my classmates were applying to colleges and taking college proficiency tests, I could not
make up my mind about a profession. My father suggested an x-ray
technology program at a local hospital. I decided to apply and was
accepted. My experience in the field of radiologic technology includes positions in nearly all the imaging modalities, as well as
teaching experience. I am currently employed as a radiology nurse.
I have found that working in radiology has been both challenging
and rewarding. My contribution to this text is an attempt to give
back some of what I have learned over the years.

I dedicate this text to the thousands of practicing radiologic and
student technologists who encounter patients every day. It is you

who can make such a difference in what our patients remember about their visits to radiology departments. Remember that patients may not always react or cooperate in the ways you think they should. Respect their individuality and privacy. It is our hope that we have given you the information you need to care for each patient, not only during examinations, but physically and emotionally as well.

KD

Preface

OUR GOAL IN WRITING THIS TEXTBOOK IS TO HELP STUDENTS in the imaging professions come to understand the importance and value of quality patient care. Some radiologic technologists do not become fully aware of their role in patient care until they actually begin their practices. In your course of study, from radiographic physics to anatomy and from patient positioning to the technical aspects of imaging procedures, it may sometimes seem that the technical is emphasized over the human, and the machine beside you is given more importance than the patient in front of you. This text is intended to help you, the student, to reach an understanding early in your education that deepens with years of experience. Because a patient is an individual human being whose interests rise above all other concerns in health care, the patient is always the focus of all health care professionals, including imaging professionals.

THE PATIENT—OUR FIRST PRIORITY

Patients are not simply bodies positioned before x-ray machines; they are feeling, thinking, unique individuals whose total well being is affected by every phase of interaction with the health care system. Thus the radiologic technologist's ability to communicate with patients, respect and advocate their rights, and provide for their safety is just as important as what may be considered the more "medical" aspects of practice.

Patient care is a dimension of radiographic practice that affects everything we do. When we are with patients, we represent the health care team in all of our actions, and we are responsible for assisting patients in meeting all of their needs. For example, we practice infection control techniques not only to protect the patient we are treating but all others in the health care setting as well. We continually assess patients' conditions to ensure continuous quality patient care. We understand the circumstances of patients with catheters or vascular access devices or who are receiving medications; we can adjust our techniques as needed in patients' best interests. These are just a few of the ways we integrate patient care into our daily practice.

These topics are covered in this text, and they include all the patient care responsibilities in the scope of practice for imaging professionals. *Integrated patient care* is the key phrase in the title of this text and is a primary theme throughout—high-quality patient care is essential in everything we do.

CONTENT AND ORGANIZATION

We have tried to consistently focus on the real world—what the radiologic technologist really needs to know for quality practice, including appropriate backgrounds and theoretical explanations to help explain and clarify these realities. Similarly, we used a writing style that is clear and to-the-point and directs the reader to the essentials. The full-color photographs and illustrations also help create a bridge from the concepts to the implications and applications of patient care in everyday practice.

After all the imaging professions are introduced in the first chapter, information related to each profession is included throughout the text whenever relevant. Information on the different levels of basic human needs is also integrated. In addition, the importance of communicating with patients also is echoed in the different contexts of patient care provided.

LEARNING AIDS

The specific features and formats used in this text are also designed to help you focus on and retain key information. The objectives that open each chapter immediately direct your attention to the essential content within the chapter and help you organize your studies. The listing of key terms for the chapter, which are in bold when they are first defined in the text, assist you with learning the new language and concepts of radiography. Study questions at the end of each chapter help you to assess your understanding of the information and ability to meet the chapter objectives, as well as prepare for your future registry examination. Step-by-step procedures including illustrations of all key steps help you learn new procedures more easily and ensure correct performance of techniques. Special display boxes and tables highlight important information for quick reference. In all, we have chosen to use the features and formats that are effective for student-centered learning. It is for you, the student who is reading and studying this material independently in the context of a course of instruction, that we designed this text.

ANCILLARIES

For the instructor, we have provided a slide set and Instructor's Manual with additional resources to supplement class discussions, including lab exercises and test questions.

As you read the words and look at the illustrations on these pages, we hope you always see a patient—a real person. There is a cartoon in a medical journal of a crotchety old radiologist viewing a chest x-ray. A patient inadvertantly steps between the radiologist and the radiograph, momentarily blocking the radiologist's view. As the radiologist is reaching out to push the patient out of the way, he is saying, "Excuse me, but I can't see my patient!" How true and how sad this cartoon is, for in focusing only on the x-ray, the radiologist is missing the real patient right before his eyes. We hope this text will help you keep you focused on the patient throughout your education and into your practice.

NINA KOWALCZYK
KATHLEEN DONNETT

Acknowledgments

THE CREATION OF THIS TEXT WAS VERY TIME-CONSUMING, AND the support we received from many sources was invaluable. Most important, we would like to thank our spouses Doug and Ron, for their love, encouragement, and unending support. We would also like to thank our children, Nick, Erin, and Alex, for sharing their love of life and learning. Our sincerest gratitude is also extended to our editors, Jeanne Rowland and Tom Lochhaas, for keeping us on track when we really wanted to take a break! Our thanks also to Pat Watson (our photographer), Riverside Methodist Hospitals, and all who helped with the photo shoot marathon: Michele Diesen, Eileen Buckholz, Mercedes Delaserda, Ashok Saraswat, Tim Mills, Larry Martin, Rome and Angel Wadligton, Nicholas and Daniel Evans, Tina Varro, Staci Jamison, Julie Tanner, Kay Sadowski, Barbara Kinsey, and Erin Donnett. Thanks also to The Ohio State University Hospitals Department of Radiology and the many other friends and colleagues who have supported and inspired us throughout this endeavor.

Reviewers

MICHAEL BLOYD, RT, RN
Director of Educational Services,
Taylor County Hospital,
Campbellsville, Kentucky

MARYELLEN BRAZZELL, BS, RT(R), ARRT
Program Director,
Marian Health Center,
School of Radiologic Technology,
Sioux City, Iowa

JOLENE CARSON, MA, RT(R), FASRT
Cardiology Services Director,
Glenwood Regional Medical Center,
West Monroe, Louisiana

KENNETH GEORGE, BA, RT(R)
Assistant Professor and Vice-Chairperson,
Medical Radiography,
SUNY Health Science Center,
Syracuse, New York

LYNN HANKS, RT(R)(M)
Kennestone Hospital,
Marietta, Georgia

GEORGE HEISER, RT(R)
Program Director,
Brandywine Hospital,
School of Radiologic Technology,
Coatesville, Pennsylvania

PATRICIA HOCHSTUHL, BS, RT(R)
Clinical Instructor,
Cooperative Radiography Program,
Memorial Hospital of Burlington County,
Mt. Holly, New Jersey

DARRELL McKAY, PhD, RT(R), FASRT
Department Chair;
Professor of Radiologic Science,
St. Louis Community College,
St. Louis, Missouri

MARY ELLEN NEWTON, RT(R)(M)
Clinical Instructor,
School of Radiology,
St. Francis Hospital,
Evanston, Illinois

BETTY PALMER, RT(R)
Director, Radiologic Sciences,
Portland Community College,
Portland, Oregon

ANGELA PICKWICK, MS, RT(R)
Program Coordinator,
Department of Radiologic Technology,
Montgomery College,
Takoma Park, Maryland

JANE SHAW, BA, RT(R)
Instructor, Allied Health Department,
Radiography Program,
Community College of Rhode Island,
Lincoln, Rhode Island

ANDREW WOODWARD, MA, RT(R)
Department Head, Radiologic Technology,
WOR-WIC Community College,
Salisbury, Maryland

Contents

Integrated Patient Care
for the
Imaging Professional

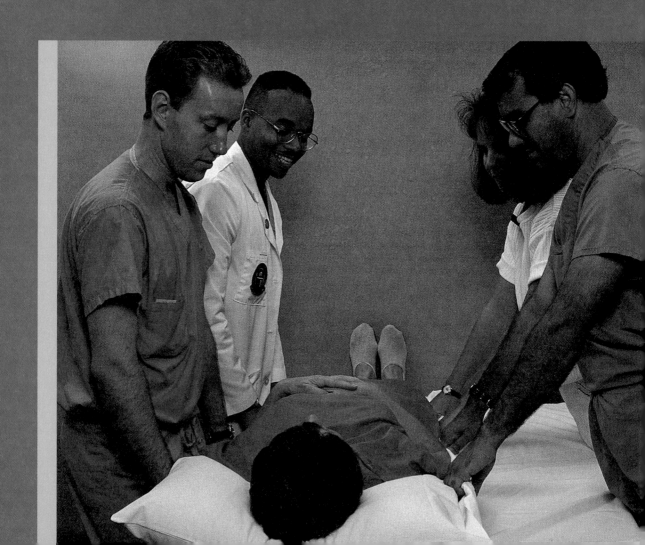

Introduction to the Profession

Key Terms

Contents

HISTORICAL PERSPECTIVE

EDUCATIONAL REQUIREMENTS

ACCREDITATION AND CERTIFICATION

    EDUCATIONAL PROGRAMS

    CERTIFYING ORGANIZATIONS

    HEALTH CARE REGULATORY AGENCIES

CONTINUING EDUCATION

PROFESSIONAL ORGANIZATIONS

CAREER OPPORTUNITIES AND PRACTICE SETTINGS

THE HEALTH CARE TEAM

THE HEALTH-ILLNESS CONTINUUM

THE HEALTH CARE DELIVERY SYSTEM

    ECONOMIC FACTORS AFFECTING HEALTH CARE DELIVERY

    REIMBURSEMENT PLANS

Objectives

AFTER COMPLETING THIS CHAPTER, THE STUDENT WILL BE ABLE TO:

1. Briefly explain the history of radiologic technology.
2. Describe the various types of educational programs for radiographers, nuclear medicine technologists, radiation therapy technologists, and diagnostic medical sonographers.
3. Specify the various accrediting organizations for educational programs and health care institutions.

4. Differentiate between certification and licensure for radiologic technologists.
5. Identify various career opportunities available for radiologic technologists.
6. Describe the professional groups that help make up the health care team.
7. Explain the concept of the health-illness continuum.
8. Demonstrate a working knowledge of current changes in the health care delivery system.

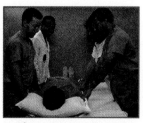

WELCOME TO THE FIELD OF MEDICAL imaging and a career that is fulfilling, challenging, and changing. Whether you plan a career in radiography, diagnostic medical sonography, nuclear medicine technology, radiation oncology, or a subspecialty of any of these fields, the concepts discussed in this text are important for you.

Imaging professionals provide a wide range of services, using technology founded on theoretical knowledge and scientific concepts. As a radiologic technologist, you will operate sophisticated imaging equipment, critique images, and make independent judgments and decisions daily. You will not just be a caregiver, you will be a patient advocate and educator as well—a person who always respects the dignity of the patient.

HISTORICAL PERSPECTIVE

The field of radiologic technology originated with the discovery of **x-rays** in 1895 by Wilhelm Konrad Röntgen, a German physicist. Röntgen chose the mathematical symbol x to name the mysterious rays because it represents the unknown. Röntgen knew that his discovery would change the world of science and medicine. He received the first Nobel Prize in Physics in 1901 for his discovery of and research involving x-rays.

Röntgen's discovery led to the development of modern techniques in radiology that are practiced today. The use of x-rays in the United States reportedly began at Dartmouth College in February 1896.

Radiology has developed considerably over the past century. Advances in radiologic equipment such as image receptors, automatic film processors, transistors, and computers, as well as the development of certain drugs and other pharmaceuticals, have paved the way for current radiologic technology. These advances have led to the development of imaging subspecialties such as cardiovascular-interventional procedures, computed tomography, magnetic resonance imaging, computed radiography, mammography, and diagnostic medical sonography. These subspecialties are described later in this chapter.

EDUCATIONAL REQUIREMENTS

The roles and responsibilities of imaging professionals have grown and expanded to keep up with changes in technology. Educational programs have developed and evolved to meet the requirements of the various specializations. Each specialty requires formal education and certification. Licensing and certification for each modality help ensure quality care for all patients.

There are three types of radiography programs: (1) a 2-year certificate program, (2) a 2-year associate degree program, and (3) a 4-year baccalaureate degree program. A graduate of any of these programs can practice as a radiographer. Careers in radiologic education and management generally require a baccalaureate degree.

Educational programs for other imaging professions, such as nuclear medicine technology, radiation oncology, and diagnostic medical sonography, vary from 1 to 2 years. The length of each program depends on the prerequisite knowledge required for the specific program. In most cases a radiographer can complete the additional necessary education in 1 year. Some sonography programs accept students who are not radiographers and require 2 years of education.

ACCREDITATION AND CERTIFICATION

The accreditation of educational programs helps ensure that the educational institutions follow an established curriculum based on sound scientific principles and a dedication to high-quality patient care.

EDUCATIONAL PROGRAMS

Educational programs in radiography must be accredited by and comply with basic educational standards set by the Joint Review Committee on Education in Radiologic Technology (JRCERT). This committee was established in 1969 and has since become an independent accrediting agency. Educational programs in nuclear medicine technology must be accredited by the Joint Review Committee on Education in Nuclear Medicine Technology (JRCNMT), which was established in 1970. In sonography, educational programs must be accredited by the Joint Review Committee on Education in Diagnostic Medical Sonography (JRCDMS), which was established in 1979.

All of these educational programs, regardless of their specialties, must follow guidelines outlined by the appropriate Joint Review Committee in "The Essentials of an Accredited Program." This document specifies the way educational programs must operate to obtain and maintain accreditation. Both classroom and clinical education are crucial for students because expertise in the imaging technologies is a result of theoretical knowledge and clinical practice.

CERTIFYING ORGANIZATIONS

After graduation, you are eligible to take the certification examination for your field or specialty. Certification represents competency in your profession. In diagnostic radiology departments this translates into quality patient care, good radiation safety practices, diagnostic quality radiographs, and cost-effective and efficient imaging operations.

Various agencies grant certification in the radiologic sciences. Many states require certification to obtain a license to practice. A license differs from certification in that a license is granted by the state. About three fourths of the states have licensing laws covering the practice of radiologic technology.

The largest certifying organization in medical imaging is the American Registry of Radiologic Technologists (ARRT). The ARRT, established in 1922, was incorporated in 1936 as the American Registry of X-Ray Technicians. In 1962 the registry developed examinations for certification in nuclear medicine technology and radiation therapy technology, and the name was changed to its present name. In 1977 the title *radiologic technologist* was adopted in place of "x-ray technologist."

On successful completion of the examination, individuals are registered with the ARRT and may use the title registered technologist (RT). The technologist's specific specialty is designated as radiography (R), nuclear medicine (N), or radiation therapy (T).

Certified radiographers may take subspecialty examinations in cardiovascular-interventional technology (CV) or mammography (M). The ARRT is developing subspecialty examinations in computed tomography, magnetic resonance imaging, and quality assurance/quality control.

Nuclear medicine technologists may also obtain certification through the Nuclear Medicine Technology Certification Board (NMTCB). Successful completion of this examination earns the title certified nuclear medicine technologist (CNMT).

Certification for diagnostic medical sonographers is granted by the American Registry of Diagnostic Medical Sonographers (ARDMS). The ARDMS was founded in 1975 to certify individuals specializing in one of the three subspecialties in sonography. On successful completion of the examination the individual earns the title registered diagnostic medical sonographer (RDMS), registered diagnostic cardiac sonographer (RDCS), or registered vascular technologist (RVT).

Each of the certifying organizations described requires annual fees, adherence to specific ethical standards, and continuing education to remain in good standing. The theoretical concepts in each field, which are covered in the certifying examinations, form the necessary base of knowledge needed to practice current technology and to develop professional autonomy and accountability.

HEALTH CARE REGULATORY AGENCIES

Just as educational institutions must meet certain standards, so must health care facilities. They are subject to a variety of regulating agencies, including the Joint Commission on Accreditation of Health Care Organizations (JCAHO), state health departments, the Occupational Safety and Health Administration (OSHA), the Food and Drug Administration (FDA), and the Nuclear Regulatory Commission (NRC). Compliance with some agencies, such as the JCAHO, is voluntary, whereas compliance with other agencies, such as OSHA, is mandatory.

CONTINUING EDUCATION

Since its inception, the ARDMS has required continuing education for technologists to renew their certification and remain in good professional standing. More recently the ARRT also began requiring continuing education for certification renewal. Because radiologic technology is a dynamic profession, continuing education is needed to maintain competence. All technologists must keep their knowledge, theories, and clinical skills up-to-date.

Continuing education involves formal, organized teaching programs designed to improve and maintain the quality of practice of medical imaging. Continuing education is offered by professional organizations, educational institutions, and in-service education programs provided by employers. These programs help technologists remain informed about new developments in today's highly technical and ever-changing health care delivery system.

PROFESSIONAL ORGANIZATIONS

Radiologic technology is more than a collection of specific tasks or skills, it is a profession. A professional is conscientious when providing a specific service and is knowledgeable about the field and all areas of practice. As a professional, you are responsible and accountable for your actions toward others as well as yourself. An important aspect of professionalism is active participation in professional organizations.

Professional organizations provide opportunities for continuing education and encourage networking and communication with other imaging professionals within the community, state, country, and world. Students have the opportunity to become involved with professional organizations early in their educational programs, since local and state societies offer many social and educational activities for students as well as technologists.

The American Society of Radiologic Technologists (ASRT) is the largest national radiologic professional organization and represents all imaging modalities. It was established in 1920 to advance the profession of radiologic technology and promote high standards of education and patient care. The ASRT is the primary policy maker in the field of radiologic technology. Among its many benefits for members are continuing education opportunities and a bimonthly professional journal, *Radiologic Technology*.

Every state has a society affiliated with the ASRT. Each state society appoints two delegates to sit in the ASRT's House of Delegates; each ASRT region also elects 10 chapter delegates from specific disciplines of practice (radiation therapy, sonography, nuclear medicine, mammography, and so on) to sit in the house. The ASRT House of Delegates is the primary voice of the radiologic profession and makes decisions that affect imaging technologies. State societies maintain affiliate local societies that represent cities or regions within each state. In addition to state societies, the International Society of Radiographers and Radiologic Technologists (ISRRT) was established in 1959 and is an international organization of radiologic professionals.

During the years, other professional societies have evolved to meet the needs of specific imaging modalities or areas of practice. These include the American Healthcare Radiology Administrators (AHRA), the Association of Educators in Radiologic Sciences (AERS), the Society of Diagnostic Medical Sonographers (SDMS), the Society of Nuclear Medicine (SNM), and the Society for Magnetic Resonance Imaging (SMRI). These organizations all provide continuing education opportunities and help advance the radiologic sciences.

CAREER OPPORTUNITIES AND PRACTICE SETTINGS

The settings in which radiologic technologists practice have changed over the years. In the past most technologists worked in hospitals and had very defined roles within the radiology department. Current trends in health care have expanded technologists' duties in the hospital and outpatient settings as well. Many institutions now cross-train technologists so that they can assume additional patient care tasks. These tasks may include assisting with general patient care, phlebotomies, and electrocardiograms.

Most radiologic technologists are employed in hospitals. Often the hospital radiology department encompasses a variety of imaging modalities. General diagnostic radiology includes both **radiographic image** (static image) production, such as chest and skeletal x-rays, and **fluoroscopic imaging** (dynamic imaging), such as barium studies and myelography. Radiographers perform studies in the operating room, emergency department, and patient rooms using mobile x-ray equipment (Fig. 1-1).

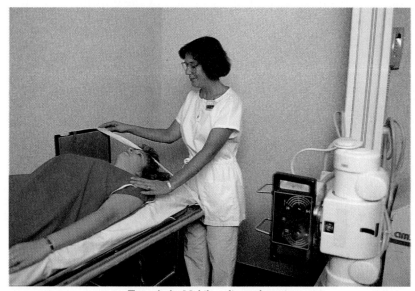

FIG. 1-1 Mobile radiography unit.

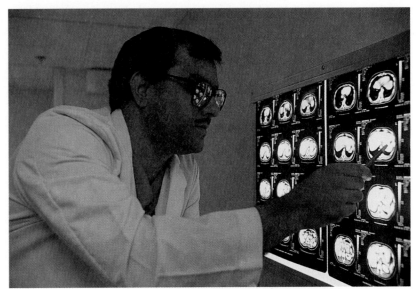

FIG. 1-2 Images produced by computed tomography.

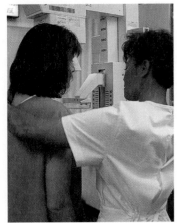

FIG. 1-3
Mammography.

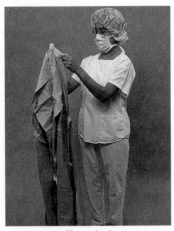

FIG. 1-4
In the cardiovascular-interventional
radiography area of the radiology
department, as in surgical areas,
the technologist maintains
sterile conditions.

Computed tomography (CT) uses highly specialized x-ray equipment to produce cross-sectional images of the body (Fig. 1-2). The equipment consists of a detector and fine x-ray beam that are enclosed in a housing called a *gantry*. The computer-generated images that are produced are much more revealing than general radiographs.

Mammography is radiography of the breast (Fig. 1-3). It has become an area of specialization as a result of the growing awareness of breast cancer and mammography's important role in early cancer detection. Mammography is used to screen patients without symptoms, diagnose patients with symptoms, localize masses before surgery, and perform core needle–biopsy procedures of the breast. Mammography departments must meet strict federal government guidelines on image production, credentialing of staff, quality assurance, and results reporting.

Cardiovascular-interventional radiography involves both diagnostic imaging and therapeutic intervention. Diagnostic studies use catheters and special medications called *contrast materials* to visualize the heart and blood vessels in the body. Therapeutic techniques include venous filtering to prevent blood clots from reaching the lungs, stenting to maintain patency of a vessel after balloon dilatation, and inserting drainage tubes. This specialty area is similar to a small operating suite within the radiology department (Fig. 1-4) and requires highly specialized equipment and a specialized health care team.

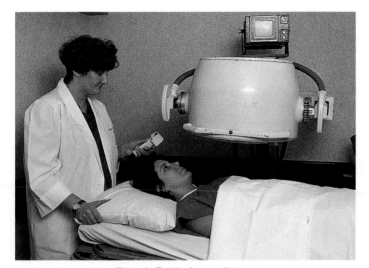

FIG. 1-5 Nuclear medicine.

Radiation therapy (or **radiation oncology**) is not used to diagnose disease but to treat disease. The diseased part of the patient's body is exposed to various types of high-level radiation while healthy areas are protected and maintained. Radiation therapy is often used to treat malignant diseases such as cancer. It may be used alone or in combination with surgery or chemotherapy.

Nuclear medicine uses radioactive isotopes or radiopharmaceuticals. Unlike the areas of radiology described previously, nuclear medicine equipment does not emit radiation. Instead, it acts like a camera by detecting radiation emitted by substances in the patient (Fig. 1-5) and producing an image. Because the results of nuclear medicine procedures provide important information about the physiologic function of organs and systems, they are used to diagnose and treat various diseases.

Diagnostic medical sonography, or **ultrasound,** uses sound waves to produce images of structures within the body. Sound waves are produced by a specialized crystal that is in a device called a *transducer*. The transducer listens to the return echoes from the sound waves, and the information is processed by a computer. The images produced are similar to those produced by sonar, which uses similar methods to aid in ship navigation. Because ultrasound does not use ionizing radiation, it is commonly used in obstetrics and gynecology procedures such as visualization of the fetus in the uterus (Fig. 1-6).

Magnetic resonance imaging (MRI) is another imaging procedure that does not use ionizing radiation. MRI produces images with a large, supercooled electromagnet and radio waves (Fig. 1-7). Like CT, MRI produces sectional and three-dimensional computer-generated images. MRI provides both anatomic and physiologic information for disease diagnosis.

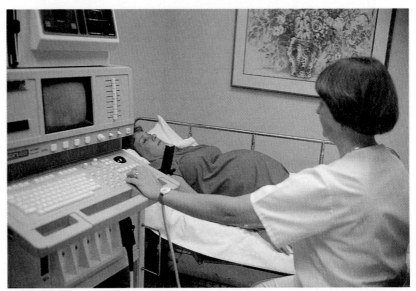

FIG. 1-6 Ultrasound.

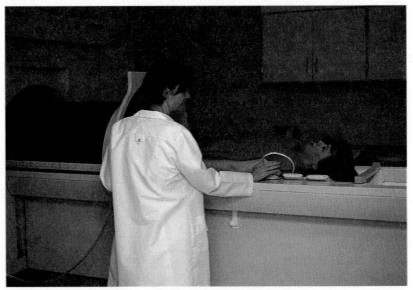

FIG. 1-7 Magnetic resonance imaging.

In addition to the specializations discussed, radiologic technologists have career opportunities in related areas, such as radiology management, hospital administration, education, clinical research, quality assurance, health physics, commercial sales, and commercial applications. Technologists may be employed in physicians' offices, outpatient imaging centers, mobile imaging companies, educational institutions, governmental agencies, and equipment or pharmaceutical companies.

THE HEALTH CARE TEAM

In patient care settings such as hospitals, clinics, and outpatient imaging centers, technologists work with other health care professionals to provide total health care for patients and their families. The health care team is composed of physicians, nurses, allied health professionals, and other specialists such as social workers and clergy (Fig. 1-8).

A **physician** is an individual who has earned a doctor of medicine (MD) degree or a doctor of osteopathy (DO) degree. Physicians must complete postgraduate training as interns and residents and must pass a licensing examination before they can practice medicine. Some physicians specialize in specific areas within medicine or surgery, and others work as generalists or family prac-

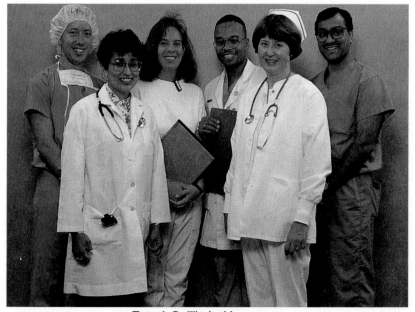

FIG. 1-8 The health care team.

titioners. A **radiologist** is a physician who specializes in the performance and interpretation of radiologic procedures.

A **registered nurse** (RN) is an individual who has graduated from an accredited nursing program and has passed a licensing examination. Nurses are generally primary caregivers, and they interact with all members of the health care team. Nurses perform a variety of functions within health care settings. Because they are patient advocates as well as direct patient caregivers, they promote the best interests of patients and defend their rights. Clinical nurse specialists (CNSs) hold a graduate degree in nursing and have expertise in a specialized area such as cancer, cardiovascular disease, or pediatrics. Nurses may also serve as anesthetists, nurse practitioners, or midwives.

In most hospitals, registered nurses are assisted with direct patient care duties by licensed practical nurses (LPNs), certified medical assistants, or patient care technicians. These individuals assist in the daily bathing, feeding, and monitoring of inpatients or with obtaining medical histories and vital signs of outpatients.

Allied health care professionals include respiratory therapists (RRTs), occupational therapists (OTs), physical therapists (PTs), medical technologists (MTs), speech pathologists, and pharmacists, as well as various laboratory, orthopedic, and operating room technical personnel. Each profession plays a vital role in providing specialized services to patients and their families.

Social workers and clergy are trained to counsel patients and their families. Their duties include providing emotional support, arranging placement in long-term care facilities, and locating financial resources. Social workers, physicians, and nurses work together to develop a health care plan for each patient.

THE HEALTH-ILLNESS CONTINUUM

The World Health Organization defines health as "a state of complete physical, mental, and social well-being, not merely the absence of disease or infirmity." Although many people view health as simply the opposite of disease, there is actually an entire range of wellness between these two extremes called the **health-illness continuum.** Not all of today's health consumers think of their health in terms of this continuum (Fig. 1-9) or view their health as a dynamic state, but an individual's health changes continuously. It adapts to alterations in the environment to maintain a state of physical, emotional, social, and spiritual well-being. Neither health nor illness is an absolute state.

The health care professional's ideas of health or wellness may

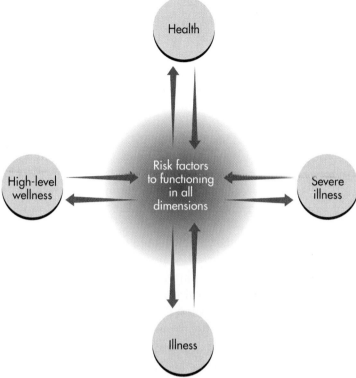

FIG. 1-9 The health-illness continuum, which ranges from high-level wellness to severe illness, provides a way to identify a patient's level of health.

differ from the patient's. Reactions to and attitudes toward illness vary from person to person depending on individual lifestyle, cultural and spiritual beliefs, and psychosocial status. Patients' assessment of their own health relates directly to individual attitudes toward health and wellness and to values and perceptions of well-being.

Health care professionals should advocate health promotion and illness prevention. For the past decade, prevention has been emphasized more than merely providing care for patients after they have become ill. True preventive care, or primary prevention, is given before disease occurs while individuals are physically and mentally healthy. Preventive care is also appropriate when an individual has developed an illness and is at risk of additional complications associated with the disease. This is often called *secondary prevention*. Health care professionals can help reduce overall health care costs by practicing preventive care and promoting healthy lifestyles. For example, advocating screening mammograms can lead to early detection of cancer in asymptomatic women and results in higher patient survival rates.

THE HEALTH CARE DELIVERY SYSTEM

Health care delivery has changed dramatically in recent years. The hospital was once the major setting for health care. Patients came to hospitals for diagnosis and treatment and often stayed until they were almost fully recovered. This is no longer true. Today treatment often occurs in outpatient situations, and most patients who are admitted to hospitals are already very ill. A hospital's goal is to provide the highest quality patient care in the most efficient and cost-effective manner, so many patients are routinely discharged before they have recovered. Although some may return home, others may enter extended care facilities that provide intermediate nursing care.

In the past, medical care was evaluated on the basis of safety and efficacy. Safety factors consisted of possible side effects or complications associated with procedures or treatments. Efficacy was based on how successful medical treatments were when performed under ideal conditions established through clinical trials.

Two additional criteria, effectiveness and efficiency, are used to evaluate today's medical care. Effectiveness measures how successful medical treatments are under normal conditions rather than in controlled laboratory settings such as clinical trials. This allows measurements of a treatment's actual effect on a patient. Efficiency evaluates a particular treatment or procedure on the basis of cost and benefit. Technologic advancements in medicine force health care professionals to deal with ethical issues regarding the cost of specific interventions in relation to the actual benefits derived.

Today's health care professional should focus on the results of care, or outcomes. Aside from traditional patient outcomes such as mortality, morbidity, and complications, cost is an outcome that must also be considered. Because quality health care addresses all aspects of patient treatment, radiologic professionals should look beyond imaging procedures and examine health care delivery as a whole. Are services delivered in an appropriate time? Are the examinations that are being performed necessary? Are examinations that provide the most useful information about a patient's condition being performed? When appropriate, are certain procedures being performed on an outpatient rather than an inpatient basis to allow earlier discharge from the hospital?

Consumers of health care services have changed over the past decade. Today's knowledgeable consumers play an active role in their health care delivery. Few patients accept physician recommendations without considering the impact, benefits, and risks associated with particular treatments. Patients often seek second opinions or request that physicians outline alternatives for prescribed treatments.

ECONOMIC FACTORS AFFECTING HEALTH CARE DELIVERY

Traditional health care has been delivered using a **fee-for-service reimbursement system.** Patients receive health care without incurring direct personal expense, and health care providers have little incentive to provide cost-effective health care services. Basically, the more services rendered by a health care provider, the more money insurance companies pay that provider. This system is called a *third party payor* or *reimbursement system* because bills are paid by an insurance company or third party rather than directly by the patient.

Spiraling health care costs and concerns about access to services have led to the current focus on health care reform. Surveys in the early 1990s indicated that over three fourths of Americans believe the health care delivery system needs to be changed. It has become increasingly difficult for individuals to pay for adequate health insurance or to pay for health care services with their own resources. Health care costs have increased rapidly because of inflation and the development of new technology and expensive services. Although America has one of the most extensive health care systems in the world, it is unaffordable for many people. Therefore government agencies and private insurance companies have developed a variety of programs to help pay for health care.

In our society many people believe that access to health care is an inherent right, regardless of cultural differences or economic status. This belief led to the development of the Medicare and Medicaid programs in the 1960s. In addition, in 1965 the Social Security Act was amended to include health care coverage for the elderly and poor. Before the 1960s the government paid little attention to health care issues and had not regulated health care delivery.

In 1983 the federal government changed the system it was using to reimburse health care providers for patients receiving Medicare benefits. The **prospective reimbursement system,** which is used today, bases the government's payments for Medicare services on a **diagnostic related group (DRG) classification system.** This classification system categorizes the patient in 1 of 23 major diagnostic or disease categories according to the principal diagnosis. Each major diagnostic category, or DRG, is further divided into subcategories, resulting in a total of approximately 492 DRGs. Under this prospective reimbursement plan the government pays the hospital a set fee for each DRG classification, regardless of the actual cost of patient care. In addition, each DRG is assigned an average length of hospital stay so that health care providers will be motivated to contain costs while providing high-quality services.

REIMBURSEMENT PLANS

In 1973 the Health Maintenance Organization (HMO) Act was passed to provide comprehensive health care for individuals who voluntarily enrolled in specific, prepaid insurance plans called **health maintenance organizations.** HMOs operate under a managed care system to encourage wellness and prevent illness. Some HMOs contract with physicians and medical institutions who have agreed to provide services for a set fee to individuals enrolled in the plan. Other HMOs employ their own physicians and operate their own medical facilities.

Another insurance option offered by some companies is called a **preferred provider organization** (PPO) or an **exclusive provider organization** (EPO). A PPO or an EPO is a contractual arrangement between physicians and medical facilities and the company or insurance plan. This system provides health services at a discounted rate to individuals enrolled in the plan.

Regardless of the specific type of health care plan paying for medical services, direct reimbursements for them have declined. Health care professionals must exercise cost-containment measures to help reduce costs without sacrificing quality patient care. Cost-containment measures include using fewer diagnostic procedures, having fewer hospital admissions, and having shorter hospital stays. Health care delivery by primary care rather than specialty care physicians also helps contain costs. Many analysts believe that managed competition will lead to necessary reforms in health care. Managed competition includes a combination of market competition and competition between the managed care organizations such as HMOs, PPOs, and EPOs. Competition among providers would encourage lower prices, better management of services, more attention to patient outcomes, and an ongoing analysis of costs and benefits. Today's health care consumer wants to be able to choose health care services that are both accessible and affordable.

SUMMARY

The radiologic technology profession has grown and changed dramatically over the past decade, and further change is inevitable. The history of our profession tells us where we have been and helps us understand present practices. Your educational experience is important because it is the basis for continued learning and professional growth. Most important, the future of the profession lies in your hands, for you are the future of radiologic technology. Regardless of your specific imaging specialty and whether you devote your career to education, management, sales, or the clinical aspects of radiologic technology, you should remain active in the profession. Participate in professional societies at all levels, and commit yourself to life-long learning. Technologists who are content with the status quo will find the profession quickly passes them by.

STUDY QUESTIONS

1. When were x-rays discovered? Who is responsible for their discovery?
2. List three types of radiography educational programs.
3. Why must educational programs be accredited? Which agencies are responsible for accrediting educational programs?
4. What is the largest certifying organization in medical imaging?
5. How does participation in professional organizations enhance the practice of medical imaging?
6. List five career opportunities available to imaging professionals.
7. What four major groups of professionals make up the health care team?
8. Briefly explain the concept of the health-illness continuum.
9. Discuss current changes in the health care delivery system and the impact of these changes on both the consumer and provider.
10. Compare the various methods of reimbursement for health care services.

Two

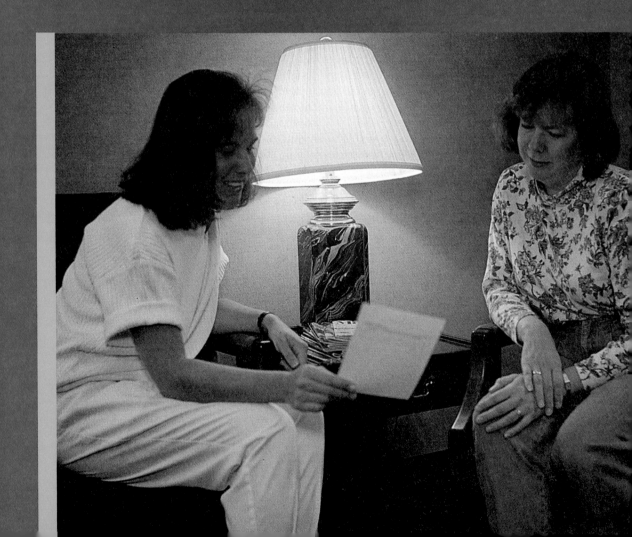

Communication

Key Terms

Contents

Objectives

AFTER COMPLETING THIS CHAPTER, THE STUDENT WILL BE ABLE TO:

1. Diagram and analyze the communication process.
2. Describe common problems that can occur in the communication process.
3. Give examples of verbal and nonverbal communication.
4. Specify three levels of communication and give examples of each level.
5. Explain the importance of personal space when communicating with others.
6. Demonstrate active listening skills.
7. Demonstrate the ability to instruct patients about imaging procedures.
8. Evaluate the role cultural diversity plays in the communication process and communicate effectively with patients from different cultures.
9. Identify common losses a patient may experience while in the hospital.
10. Specify the stages of grieving and give one example of a common behavior in each.
11. Outline a dying patient's rights.
12. Describe common problems encountered when communicating with individuals with sensory alterations.
13. Demonstrate the use of various aids to assist in communicating with individuals who have sensory deficits.
14. Explain the importance of communicating with patients with trauma or who are in a state of altered consciousness.
15. Describe the factors to consider when communicating with individuals under the influence of chemicals.
16. Describe the purpose and importance of the Americans with Disabilities Act of 1990.

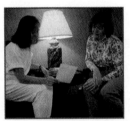

COMMUNICATION IS ONE OF THE MOST IMportant aspects of health care.

All health care professionals need effective communication skills to maintain good working relationships with patients, guests, and other health professionals. Good communication skills are not obtained automatically; you will need to work hard and be persistent to refine your skills. Many factors affect and sometimes impede effective communication (box).

Individuals who communicate well are able to completely and accurately transfer information from themselves to others. Although this seems like a straightforward process, it can be quite complex, and when ineffective, it can cause many kinds of problems. You will become a better communicator if you pay attention to the communication process while working with patients and other professionals.

FACTORS AFFECTING COMMUNICATION

- Perceptions
- Values
- Personal space
- Emotions
- Sociocultural background
- Knowledge
- Environment

THE COMMUNICATION PROCESS

A model commonly used to describe the **communication process** defines it in terms of a sender, receiver, message, and feedback (Fig. 2-1). Person A, the *sender,* begins communicating by sending a *message.* In addition to words, or verbal communication, the message includes gestures, expressions, and actions, which are all forms of **nonverbal communication.** Person B, the *receiver,* gets a message, which ideally is the same message intended by Person A. Person B responds in some way to the message, either verbally, nonverbally, or both. This response is called *feedback* because it lets Person A know what message Person B has received. If Person B gets the message exactly as intended by Person A, an accurate transfer of information has been achieved and communication has been successful. If Person B's feedback indicates that the message received was not exactly what Person A intended, Person A has the opportunity to correct the miscommunication.

Though helpful, this simple model does not demonstrate the complexity of the dynamic communication process. The receiver may not give clear feedback to the sender, for example, so the sender may incorrectly assume the receiver got the intended message. In addition, the roles of sender and receiver are not static. The

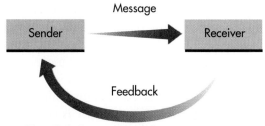

FIG. 2-1 Communication is a two-way process.

sender immediately becomes the receiver when the original receiver gives feedback. Several factors can interrupt communication and cause a person to receive an inaccurate message.

In our daily lives we do not usually analyze every step of our communication process, but we have all experienced the feeling of being misunderstood when the process breaks down. To prevent communication problems from occurring with patients, you need to become aware of the complexities of the process and refine your communication skills by paying attention to the way you communicate verbally and nonverbally.

VERBAL COMMUNICATION

Verbal communication includes spoken and written words. Communicating clearly with words may seem an elementary concept, but words have different meanings for different people and therefore are not always accurately interpreted. The way people define words is affected by their cultural background, life experiences, and education.

Some words are relative or ambiguous and can be interpreted in different ways. For example, consider the following statement: "The patient is experiencing mild flushing." This could be unclear because the word *mild* can have such a wide range of meanings. Even asking simply whether a patient is urinating frequently could result in a misunderstanding because of the ambiguity of the word *frequent.* Medical terms may also have more than one meaning. The term *decubitus* could either mean a bed sore or a patient position used in radiography. Some words may also have emotional associations that vary among persons. Which emotions do you associate with terms such as *critical, emergency,* and *cancer?* Which emotions could these terms arouse in patients?

Try to use clear, concise language when speaking to patients and other health care professionals. Effective verbal communication consists of a proper vocabulary, pacing, intonation, and clarity.

As you become more familiar with the health care field you will realize that it has its own vocabulary. Although common medical terms and phrases will become a part of your everyday vocabulary, you must remember that many of these terms are unfamiliar to patients. Avoid using complicated terminology to ensure that patients understand your message accurately. For instance, ask patients to lie on their backs rather than to lie supine. Using vocabulary patients understand is a crucial aspect of good communication.

In addition, try to speak at a speed that is comfortable for each individual patient, and pause when appropriate. *Think* about what you are going to say before you begin to speak. *Watch* the way patients react to your message to see whether you are being understood (Fig. 2-2). Speaking too quickly, especially about medical topics, may confuse some patients. Enunciate each word carefully, and try to avoid odd or prolonged pauses that may give the impression you are uncertain or uninformed or are hiding something from the patient.

Consider the common saying "It's not what you said, but how you said it." Your tone of voice expresses emotion and can have a dramatic effect on the meaning of a message. It can express a variety of feelings, from enthusiasm or disgust to concern or indifference. Although you are probably not always conscious of your tone of voice, you can learn to control it by becoming aware of the way you sound to others. Practice using a sincere, caring tone when speaking with patients and co-workers.

Overall, communicate simply, clearly, and directly. Choose your words carefully, avoid ambiguous terms, and when possible, choose simple words to express your ideas.

NONVERBAL COMMUNICATION

People communicate through gestures and actions as well as words. We may not consciously be aware of our nonverbal messages, but they are always important during face-to-face conversations. Nonverbal messages may express more than or enhance verbal messages. An action such as tapping your foot may reveal impatience, whereas pointing your finger toward people may give them the feeling that they are being accused. By being aware of what you express through your gestures and actions, you can relay a message that is consistent verbally and nonverbally and present a professional, caring image.

The way you stand, sit, and move all reflect your perception of yourself and others. Leaning forward while speaking or listening shows you are interested in and focused on the conversation. Good posture and purposeful movements communicate a professional self-assurance.

Physical appearance also sends out nonverbal messages. One of the first things another person notices about you is your appearance. As a professional, you should be a well-groomed and in appropriate attire and have good hygiene. This helps establish a sense of trust for you, the patients, and other health care workers. A sloppy appearance may indicate sloppy work habits to some patients or health care professionals. In addition, a clean and neat work environment is important because it represents your institution and your profession.

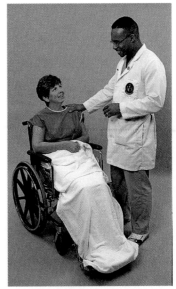

FIG. 2-2
Communicate clearly and professionally, watching the patient for verbal and nonverbal clues.

As you become aware of the way you communicate nonverbally, also pay attention to nonverbal messages conveyed by patients. Patients often express their comfort levels nonverbally rather than verbally. Be alert for *any* signs of discomfort or pain. If a patient is moving slowly because of pain, do not rush down a hall and expect the patient to be able to follow at your speed.

Facial expressions and eye contact are very strong modes of nonverbal communication. The human face can express six primary emotions: surprise, fear, anger, disgust, happiness, and sadness. Facial expressions either reinforce or contradict the verbal message, so you must be aware of this when controlling your own expressions and understanding a patient's. In our culture, maintaining eye contact while speaking with another individual communicates respect and a willingness to listen. A lack of eye contact may signal distrust, anxiety, or a lack of confidence. However, eye contact has different meanings in different cultures. In some cultures, for example, a lack of eye contact indicates a respect of authority and status.

Touch is a powerful form of nonverbal communication that is used often in health care. Touch can express affection and provide emotional support, encouragement, and personal attention. A gesture as small as holding a frightened patient's hand can be more supportive than words. Because touching is a very personal form of communication, however, use it with care and only when the patient clearly understands and accepts it. Some individuals are uncomfortable with being touched.

LEVELS OF COMMUNICATION

Communication occurs at a variety of levels. It can be as private as internal communication (communicating with yourself) or as public as speaking to a large group.

You were cautioned previously to think about what you are going to say before you begin to speak. This type of internal communication is called **intrapersonal communication.** We communicate with ourselves on this level constantly as we decide ways to appropriately express our thoughts to others. Intrapersonal communication is important when expressing your thoughts to others because it can help you avoid common barriers to good communication. For example, in the professional health care environment, judgmental statements do not promote effective communication. You should never show your personal approval or disapproval of another person. The health care professions are "helping professions," implying an unconditional acceptance of others and a respect for individuality. Avoid giving opinions, offering false reassurance, or being defensive.

Use your intrapersonal communication skills to choose the most appropriate words possible and determine the most caring way you can convey information. Caring promotes a sense of trust, and patients must trust your professional abilities.

Communication between two people (you and a patient) or in small groups (in a patient's family) is called **interpersonal communication.** The sender-receiver-feedback model described earlier depicts this level of communication. Always try to show empathy for the patient when working with patients and their families. Empathy is the ability to personally understand or perceive patients' or family members' feelings. Empathy is based on similarities of experience or derived from shared feelings as human beings. For example, you can empathize with a patient in pain if you have experienced significant pain. Empathy seems genuine to patients unlike sympathy or pity, which can seem insincere.

In all first interactions with patients, start the interpersonal communication by introducing yourself, for example: "Good morning, Mrs. Jones, my name is Jane. I will be taking an x-ray of your chest this morning." This type of introduction lets patients become comfortable with you and shows you respect their individuality. Be sure to explain any procedure performed on a patient before it has begun, regardless of its complexity. Establishing rapport is critical for developing mutual trust. Patients should be addressed as Mr., Mrs., Ms., and so on. Do not use first names except when addressing children or patients who have asked you to use their first name. *Never* use familiar terms such as "honey" or "dear" to address patients or family members.

At some time in your professional career, you will have the opportunity to speak to a group about imaging and related health issues. This third level of communication is called *public speaking*, and although it involves skills beyond those described here, good interpersonal communication skills are the foundation for developing good public speaking skills.

PERSONAL SPACE

Communicating well also takes an individual's **personal space** into consideration. This is the distance around a person that is considered private. People become uncomfortable when strangers move into this space. Because your daily work in an imaging department requires you to come into close physical contact with patients, personal space plays an important role in your profession. Be aware of the way you affect patients when you must enter their personal space. Act professionally and work to maintain effective communication. Except when absolutely necessary, keep an appropriate distance from patients and families.

A **social distance** is a distance of 4 to 12 feet between people. This is the most common and comfortable distance maintained among people working together when they are not sharing personal thoughts and feelings.

A **personal distance** is the distance between people in most face-to-face communications. Personal distance is usually a distance of 18 inches to 4 feet. Use this distance when you initially begin communicating with a patient. Introduce yourself as described earlier. Use a gentle, caring tone, but maintain a personal distance so patients will feel comfortable and confident. Gradually you can decrease the distance between you and the patient.

An **intimate distance** is a distance of 18 inches or less between people. As a technologist, you must interact within this distance when performing necessary imaging procedures. Because many patients will initially be uncomfortable having you extremely close, begin by interacting at social and personal distances before moving into an intimate distance.

Before performing a procedure, explain it to the patient. Patients must understand that you need to touch them to position them correctly. Ask permission before touching patients, and encourage them to tell you of any discomfort. Always preserve patients' autonomy by allowing them to make decisions for themselves and act independently. If patients can stand and move without assistance, encourage them to do so. Respect patients' independence and encourage self-direction.

LISTENING SKILLS

In any health care setting, most of your communication time involves listening. You can learn and practice listening skills to promote effective communication. Be attentive to others when they are speaking, and concentrate on what patients are saying. Consider the patient's needs and try to show empathy. Listen to the whole message before responding appropriately; you cannot listen if you are talking or thinking about your response. Avoid interrupting patients unless you need immediate clarification. Lean forward, maintain good eye contact, and nod when appropriate. Focus on one thought at a time. Use patients' nonverbal signals to confirm that you have received the message correctly.

Learn to be comfortable with silence. It gives you the opportunity to observe patients closely, and it can help both you and your patients organize your thoughts. Intrapersonal communication, or thinking to yourself during a moment of silence, can enhance your interpersonal communication. Do not rush the communication process. Allow patients time to express themselves completely.

When responding to patients, use language suited to their base of knowledge, education, and experience. Do not be condescending, but do not use lofty, technical language they cannot comprehend. Restate their message in your own words so that patients will know they have been understood.

PATIENT EDUCATION

As a technologist, you specialize in performing various imaging procedures. Your responsibilities include educating patients and other health professionals about these examinations. **Patient education** requires effective interpersonal communication skills for presenting information clearly and concisely.

You can often educate patients using written or audiovisual materials (Fig. 2-3). Patient education materials are available from many sources, including commercial vendors, nonprofit health organizations, professional organizations, medical "help" lines, and your own medical facility. When you show these materials to patients, however, you should explain the procedure verbally as well. Be aware that some patients may not admit they cannot read even when you hand them written materials.

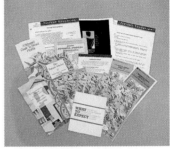

FIG. 2-3
Most facilities have materials available for patient education.

Encourage patients to ask questions about any aspect of a procedure. Answer using simple terms at age and cognitive levels appropriate for the patient. Pay attention to verbal and nonverbal feedback to ensure the patient understands your explanations.

Several medical institutions have a patient education channel on closed-circuit television for inpatients (patients who are checked into the hospital). This can be an effective way to provide patient education on a variety of imaging procedures, although patients may still have unanswered questions. Obviously, this method can only be used with patients in the hospital, and because of changes in health care delivery systems, many procedures are now performed on an outpatient basis. In most medical facilities, more than half of all imaging procedures are performed on outpatients. Therefore other methods of patient education, including the explanations you give directly to the patient, are essential.

Many institutions do not employ radiology nurses, so patient teaching is the responsibility of radiologic technologists. Most of the patient education you provide consists of instructing patients on preparing for an imaging procedure, explaining the procedure itself, or giving postprocedure instructions. Postexamination patient education may include instructions on eliminating residual barium sulfate after a gastrointestinal (GI) examination or watching for the signs and symptoms of infection after an arthrogram.

Patients must give their **informed consent** to undergo invasive procedures in which a drug, radiation, or an instrument "invades" the body. Informed consent is given after the patient has received all available information about the risks and benefits of the procedure in addition to any available alternatives. Although the physician has the responsibility to obtain the patients' consent, patients have the right to have all their questions answered, and you will often help these questions. (Chapter 4 discusses informed consent in more detail.)

Patients often question technologists about the results of examinations. You must explain that although you produce the diagnostic images, a radiologist interprets them and reports the results to the physician. Tell patients to speak with their doctors about the results of their procedures. Interpreting images for a diagnosis goes beyond the scope of your profession.

Patients will also ask about the ionizing radiation from the imaging equipment. Patients may, for example, ask how much radiation is used during a specific procedure. You should be informed and aware of the average radiation doses for procedures commonly performed in your institution. Most facilities have this information readily available, so give patients this information if it is requested. In addition, patients may ask about the harmful effects of radiation. Explain the benefits of the procedure in comparison with the risks, but do not try to coerce the patient into having the procedure. Patients have a right to refuse any procedure, so if a patient refuses, do not try to reverse the decision. Inform the physician that the procedure was not performed.

Your professional responsibilities include educating the public about your profession. Many patients believe, for example, that nurses perform imaging procedures, but they do not. Inform patients and the general public that as a technologist, you are well-educated in all facets of imaging technology. Because many people may not be aware of your training and expertise, you can educate them about the importance of your role in the health care team. Professional imaging associations such as the American Society of Radiologic Technologists provide information to help you educate the public about the imaging professions.

CULTURAL DIFFERENCES

As mentioned previously, a person's cultural background can affect the communication process. Your own cultural background can influence your interactions with patients, other health care team members, or health care providers. **Cultural diversity** results from socially inherited characteristics of a particular group being passed on from one generation to the next. These are often closely tied to an individual's nationality, race, language, religion, and other factors (box). Cultural characteristics are dynamic and may change from one generation to the next. American culture has shifted away from one that is dominated by a Caucasian European majority to a more diverse population characterized by many different ethnic and cultural groups (Fig. 2-4). Diverse lifestyles, such as living in a

CULTURAL DIVERSITY FACTORS

- Age
- Race
- Educational background and its value
- Sexual preference
- Ethnic origin
- Religious beliefs
- Disabilities

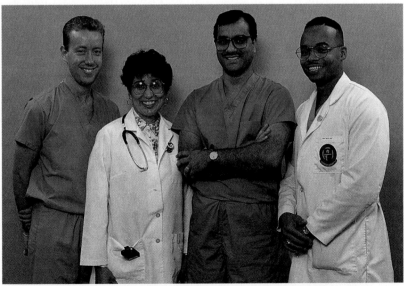

FIG. 2-4 Cultural backgrounds can influence the communication process.

single-parent home or having a blended family, add to this cultural shift and are more common today.

Understanding and working well with culturally diverse patients requires cultural literacy, which is a comfortable familiarity with many types of people and backgrounds. Explore the cultural groups in your area. While respecting peoples' cultural diversity, however, remember that we are all more alike than different. All humans strive for common goals such as the attainment of love, hope, joy, happiness, and good health. Everyone has a unique contribution to offer, so we should celebrate cultural diversity instead of viewing people from other cultures as fundamentally different. See the box for a summary of tips for communicating with patients from different cultural groups.

Cultural characteristics help shape the way people view health and illness. As a technologist, you know and are comfortable with what we consider a modern approach to health care. In some cultures, however, people better understand and are more comfortable with traditional approaches to healing. Traditional medical practices may come from ancient beliefs and folklore and include natural remedies. Almost every cultural group has some type of traditional cultural medicine. Respect patients' traditions as you practice modern medicine because as discussed earlier, a professional never judges another person's beliefs or practices.

Cultural factors can affect both nonverbal and verbal communication between you and the patient. For example, technologists may expect a patient who is in great pain to both verbalize their pain and show it in facial expressions and body movements. If the patient is from a cultural background that does not approve of physical expressions of pain, this patient may show no signs at all. Therefore technologists who assume all patients act out their pain in the same way will not be watching for different or subtle signs and important information may not be communicated.

Language is one of the most important aspects of communication that is affected by cultural diversity. If a patient does not speak

---

TIPS FOR COMMUNICATING WITH OTHER CULTURAL GROUPS

- Show respect.
- Treat all ethnic groups equally.
- Be aware of your own and the patient's nonverbal messages.
- If you do not understand something, ask for clarification.

your language, you must get an interpreter. An ideal interpreter is a family member who can translate information from you to the patient and from the patient to you. A family member may also be able to provide information about the patient's health history. If no bilingual family member is present, your institution may have its own interpreters to translate and ensure good communication between health professionals and patients. Although patients may speak a little of your language, they may not be fluent enough to completely understand everything you say. You can use your communication skills to verify patients' understanding, but get a translator if you are at all unsure whether your message has been accurately received.

SPECIAL COMMUNICATION SITUATIONS

Technologists who work in acute care settings such as hospitals and major medical centers often encounter situations that require specialized communication skills. Patients with sensory alterations, physical impairments, or mental impairments may add additional complications to the communication process. Encourage these patients to ask questions. Answer each question using simple terms appropriate to patients' comprehension levels. Remember that factors such as individual perceptions, values, emotions, culture, and educational background all play a vital role in communication.

Although special circumstances may make communication challenging, you should still try to communicate as effectively as possible.

SENSORY ALTERATIONS

Sensory deficits, sensory deprivation, and sensory overload are three types of sensory alterations. A **sensory deficit** results from defective sensory reception or perception. Blindness is a type of sensory deficit characterized by the inability to receive visual stimuli. Distorted visual stimuli may be the result of a sensory deficit caused by eye cataracts. Other sensory deficits include the inability to hear (deafness) and the inability to speak (muteness or some forms of aphasia).

Sensory deprivation results from receiving too little or low-quality stimulation. This type of sensory alteration can be caused by a physical impairment, such as a vision or hearing loss, or from being placed in isolation because of infection with a contagious disease.

Sensory overload occurs when individuals receive so much sensory stimuli that they are unable to sort out or ignore unimportant information. Individuals experiencing sensory overload cannot make sense of their perceptions of the environment. Hospitals are full of unusual sights, smells, and sounds. Although you may become accustomed to the sight of blood, the smell of urine, and the sounds of equipment being used, these same sensory stimuli can overwhelm patients and make it more difficult for individuals to cope with hospitalization.

You will undoubtedly encounter individuals with preexisting sensory alterations whether they are inpatients or outpatients. You can use the communication techniques described in this chapter with both types of patients, but the skills are especially pertinent for inpatients.

Hospital admission frightens most people. Hospitalization makes it difficult for individuals to fulfill their most basic needs (as described in Maslow's hierarchy in Chapter 6). Attaining something as basic as safety or security or as complex as self-esteem can be difficult because of illness and loss of control over daily activities.

Some patients develop temporary or permanent sensory alterations because of medical or surgical interventions while in the hospital. For example, patients may lose their ability to speak after receiving an artificial airway. Sensory alterations that inhibit communication can make patients feel isolated and insecure and can lower their self-esteem. Identify patients in these special situations and provide adequate support.

A sudden sensory loss or alteration, especially in an unfamiliar environment, can cause fear, anger, and feelings of helplessness. Health care practitioners must help patients experiencing this find alternative ways to function safely within the hospital environment.

For example, patients with visual impairments need assistance in the unfamiliar imaging department. Assist these patients by describing where you are going as you physically guide them through the department. Remove obstacles from their path, explain all procedures in detail, and never leave them standing alone in the department. Try to put patients at ease regardless of whether the procedure is performed in the imaging department or patients' hospital rooms.

Patients who are at high risk for sensory alterations include older adults, which is a result of normal physiologic and lifestyle changes; patients who are immobilized because of the need for bed rest or traction; patients who are in isolation because of an infection or immunodepressed condition; and patients with endotracheal tubes and tracheostomies.

Various communication techniques can be used in special situations (box). Common communication aids include the use of pencil and paper, felt-tip markers and marker boards, communication boards with preprinted words, letters, and pictures, flash cards, and sign language. Communication with physical gestures, such as eye blinks

COMMUNICATION METHODS

PATIENTS WITH APHASIA

- Listen to and wait for the patient to communicate.
- Do not shout or speak loudly. (Hearing loss is not the problem.)
- If the patient has problems with comprehension, use simple, short questions and facial gestures to give additional clues.
- If the patient has problems speaking, ask questions that require simple yes or no answers or blinking of the eyes. Offer pictures or a communication board so that the patient can point.
- Give the patient time to understand.
- Do not pressure or tire the patient.

PATIENTS WITH AN ARTIFICIAL AIRWAY

- Use pictures, objects, or word cards so that the patient can point.
- Offer a pad and pencil or magic slate so that the patient can write messages.
- Do not speak loudly or shout.
- Provide an artificial voice box (vibrator) to help the patient with a laryngectomy to speak.

PATIENTS WITH A HEARING IMPAIRMENT

- Get the patient's attention. Do not startle the patient when entering the room. Do not approach the patient from behind. Be sure the patient knows you wish to speak.

- Face the patient. Illuminate your face and lips to promote lip reading.
- If the patient wears glasses, be sure they are clean so that your gestures and face can be seen. If the patient wears a hearing aid, make sure it is in place and working.
- Speak slowly and articulate clearly. Older adults may take longer to process verbal messages.* Use a normal tone of voice and speech inflections. Refrain from speaking with something in your mouth.
- When you are not understood, rephrase rather than repeat the information.
- Use visible aids. Speak with your hands, your face, and your eyes.
- Do not shout. Loud sounds usually have a higher pitch and may impede hearing by accentuating vowel sounds and concealing consonants.* If it is necessary to raise your voice, speak in lower tones.
- Talk toward the patient's best or normal ear.
- Use gestures or written information to enhance the spoken word.
- Do not restrict a deaf patient's hands. Never have intravenous lines in both of the patient's hands if the preferred method of communication is sign language.†

Modified from Potter PA, Perry AG: *Fundamentals of nursing: concepts, process, and practice*, ed. 3, 1993, Mosby.
*From Bernardini L: *Top Clin Nurs* 72, 1985.
†From Chovaz C: *Can Nurs* 85(3):34, 1989.

or finger movements, may be possible for simple responses such as yes and no. For patients with hearing loss, act out simple instructions in an exaggerated way.

Individuals with sensory deficits often develop their own alternative means of communication. Observe patients for cues, and remember that deficits do not affect their intellectual abilities. These individuals often use other sensory stimuli to enhance their communication skills. For example, a deaf or hearing-impaired patient may read lips, use sign language, use a hearing aid, or communicate by written notes. Although visually impaired patients cannot observe facial expressions or other nonverbal communication cues, they may rely on intonation and vocal inflection to detect emotional tones in a conversation. Aphasic patients may communicate with the help of communication boards or mechanical vibrators.

COMMUNICATING WITH PATIENTS WHO ARE IN A STATE OF ALTERED CONSCIOUSNESS

Individuals who have sustained trauma to the head may be in a state of altered consciousness. These patients are often combative or disoriented. Communicate with them calmly and professionally to put them at ease. Do not raise your voice, and do not become agitated. Combative individuals who place themselves or caregivers in danger may be physically restrained with soft (Fig. 2-5) or leather (Fig. 2-6) restraints. These patients should never be left alone. The restraints should not be removed unless absolutely necessary, but if they are removed, an attendant should remain with the patient at all times to prevent injury.

Explain the imaging procedure to all patients before you begin, regardless of their mental and physical status. Speak to patients normally, even if they are nonresponsive. Many health care profession-

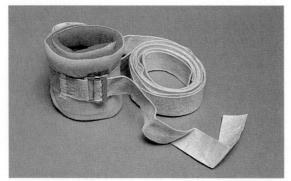

FIG. 2-5 Soft restraints.

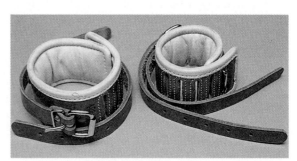

FIG. 2-6 Leather restraints.

als believe that nonresponsive and even unconscious patients may be able to receive stimuli. Hearing may be the last sense lost when patients are unconscious and the first sense regained when they are conscious. Do not discuss any matters in the presence of unconscious patients that you would not normally discuss if they were conscious.

COMMUNICATING WITH PATIENTS WHO ARE UNDER THE INFLUENCE OF CHEMICALS

Chemical dependency and substance abuse are growing problems in the United States. You may commonly encounter patients under the influence of alcohol or other drugs. Substance abuse can affect anyone, regardless of socioeconomic status, education, race, ethnic origin, gender, or occupation. Do not be judgmental and treat all patients with dignity and respect.

Alcohol and other drugs (Fig. 2-7) may be used, misused, or abused. **Drug use** is the act of taking medication as prescribed or following directions for an over-the-counter drug. **Drug misuse** is the act of taking a drug that was prescribed for someone else, not following directions for doses, or inappropriately using an over-the-counter medication. **Drug abuse** is the act of inappropriately using mood-altering chemicals, which if abused in sufficient quantities and over a sufficient length of time can cause **chemical dependency.**

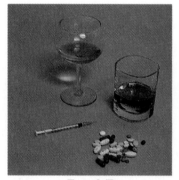

FIG. 2-7
Many different chemical substances alter consciousness.

In many cases, patients may have developed a pathologic condition such as liver disease as a result of a chemical dependency such as alcohol abuse. You may also encounter patients in the emergency room who have been injured as a result of drug abuse or have overdosed. Depending on the drug that has been abused, these patients may be disoriented, combative, or agitated. Do not raise your voice or lose patience while speaking to these patients.

The behavior of chemically dependent individuals varies depending on the type of chemical substance that has been used. Intoxicated individuals may be hostile, have impaired judgment, be uncoordinated, and have slurred speech. Amphetamine abuse may result in hyperactivity and irritability. Individuals abusing cocaine may also exhibit hyperactivity and irritability and may become easily agitated. Hallucinogen use distorts perception and results in illusions and delusions; individuals using hallucinogens may be easily agitated and can become quite violent.

Work as quickly as possible with patients who are dependent patients or under the influence of a substance, and never leave them alone in the department.

AMERICANS WITH DISABILITIES ACT

In 1990 the U.S. Congress passed the Americans with Disabilities Act (ADA) to provide comprehensive civil rights protection to individuals with disabilities. This act defines a disabled individual as one who has a physical or mental impairment that "substantially limits one or more major life activities." **Physical impairments** are any physiological disorders or conditions, including cosmetic disfigurements. **Mental impairments** include mental retardation, organic brain syndrome, emotional and mental illness, and specific learning disabilities. The physical or mental impairment limits people in one or more of the following major life activities: walking, breathing, seeing, learning, working, speaking, performing manual tasks, hearing, and caring for themselves.

The ADA affects you both as a student and as an employee. The ADA provides qualified individuals who have disabilities with equal employment opportunities. In a technologist's job description, health care institutions must include the physical requirements to perform imaging procedures, as well as job duties and functions. Educational programs must also include this information as part of the application process.

According to the ADA, qualified individuals with disabilities are individuals who can satisfy the requisite skill, education, experience, and other job-related requirements of the employment position and can perform the essential functions of the job with or without reasonable accommodations. Reasonable accommodations include modifications or adjustments to the job or work environment that enable the individual to perform essential job functions.

DEATH AND DYING

Effective communication is especially important when working with patients who are seriously ill or dying. As a technologist who works in the health care field, you will encounter patients and family members experiencing loss or coping with a terminal illness. Because you will be working with these people, you must come to terms with your own mortality and be able to cope with your emotions about death and dying.

Take the time to consider your thoughts and concerns about death and dying, which may be difficult if this is your first encounter with this delicate subject. Health professionals are often so focused on curing patients that they find it difficult to deal with death. Some health care professionals may even associate death with a failure to provide adequate care. Instead, death should be consid-

COMMON FEELINGS OF LOSS

PATIENTS MAY EXPERIENCE FEELINGS OF LOSS IN THE FOLLOWING AREAS:

- Health
- Independence/control
- Privacy
- Body image
- Self-confidence
- Financial security
- Productivity
- Normal daily routines
- Sleep
- Sexual function

ered a natural end to life. Often health care professionals can only delay death, and even the best care cannot prolong life. You need to accept these realities and deal with your own feelings so that you can give the necessary support to patients and their families.

People who experience a significant loss adapt to it gradually through a **grieving process.** This process is a sequence of responses and behaviors most people experience after a loss. Patients who learn they have a terminal illness also go through this process; they grieve for their own loss. A sense of loss causes stress and affects an individual's self-concept and self-worth. People respond in different ways to death; they may have feelings of anger, guilt, sadness, and fear. These emotions help the individual mentally cope with the loss but can lead to physical problems such as gastrointestinal disturbances, fatigue, and insomnia. Grieving is important, however, if the person is to continue living and having new insights and a direction in life. Even patients with a terminal illness can become comfortable with and accepting of their own death. (See the box for the types of loss patients may experience.)

THE GRIEVING PROCESS

The grieving process is a very personal experience. Technologists and other health professionals should be supportive of patients and families who are grieving. Understanding what patients and families are experiencing can help you be more supportive.

Dr. Elisabeth Kubler-Ross described five stages in the grieving process: (1) denial, (2) anger, (3) bargaining, (4) depression, and (5) acceptance. Both patients and family members may experience these grieving stages, but how long a person remains in any particular stage varies according to the individual. When a person experiences a significant loss, grieving may last anywhere from 6 months to 2 years. The way people grieve depends on several factors, in-

cluding their age and developmental stage, beliefs, roles, relationships, and socioeconomic status.

DENIAL

Denial is the first stage of the grieving process. Patients try to act
as if there is nothing wrong. They do not acknowledge the loss or
illness and either do not want to or cannot deal with treatment decisions. At this stage, people typically believe that although others
may experience this loss, they will not.

ANGER

The second stage of the grieving process is **anger.** Patients resist
their feelings of loss. These patients or family members may act out
their anger and strike out at others. Knowing the meaning of this
type of behavior will help you deal with it more effectively. If a patient or family member becomes angry with you, do not take it personally. The person is progressing through the grieving process,
and this reaction is normal.

BARGAINING

Bargaining is the third stage of the grieving process. During this
stage, patients or family members postpone accepting the reality of
the situation. They often become very open to suggestions for medical treatment and believe that if they act appropriately, they will be
spared the impending loss. They may also feel guilty about their
previous outbursts of anger.

DEPRESSION

The fourth stage of the grieving process is **depression.** Patients finally realize the loss is a permanent reality, and they become very
aware of the force of its impact in their lives. They typically feel de-
pressed and lonely, and they mourn the loss. Patients or family
members often become withdrawn. Offering your silent support
may be the best way to deal with someone who is in this stage.

ACCEPTANCE

The final grieving stage is **acceptance.** In this stage, patients begin
to deal with the loss. Patients who have experienced losses that
do not involve death may now accept rehabilitation. Patients who
accept that they have a terminal illness begin to deal with their
pain and awareness of mortality. At this point, patients or family
members may want to openly discuss the illness and impend-

ing death. You should be open with them and not give false reassurances.

COMMUNICATION ISSUES

In situations involving a loss, do not forget that patients and family members are grieving or you may block effective communication. You should feel comfortable talking about feelings and not avoid discussions about the loss. Be open to talking about anything dying patients want to discuss. These conversations help patients maintain good self-esteem as well as a sense of identity and dignity. Terminally ill patients sometimes have particular odors or may be confused or combative. Unfortunately, patients may be avoided by others because of factors like these. These patients may feel isolated and have more difficulty grieving and accepting their loss. You can help by simply listening and providing comfort and support.

Terminally ill patients often have experiences that threaten their dignity. Continue to maintain confidentiality. Use your communication skills to encourage patients and family members to express their feelings and clarify their thoughts about their loss. Being a good listener can help them work through their feelings and accept death. Although you may not know these patients as well as other health care professionals, consider their needs and be as helpful as you can by acting in a mature, professional manner.

DYING PATIENTS' RIGHTS

The rights of dying patients are described in the box. One key right is the right to choose the location for care. Although some patients may choose to be in an acute care hospital, another patients may prefer to stay at home in a more familiar environment. Hospice care is one alternative for patients who prefer home care.

Hospice care for terminally ill patients focuses on family centered care. Instead of trying to cure the illness when there is no real hope of improvement, palliative treatment—treatment to make patients feel more comfortable—is emphasized. Family members usually serve as the major caregivers in hospice care, but they are assisted by physicians, nurses, clergy, social workers, and specially trained volunteers. The goal of hospice care is to help patients enjoy time they have remaining as fully as possible in the home or a home-like environment. After the patient's death the hospice team continues to help family members deal with their bereavement. The hospice approach to health care effectively manages the illness, death, and needs of the family.

THE DYING PERSON'S BILL OF RIGHTS

I have the right to be treated as a living human being until I die.

I have the right to maintain a sense of hopefulness, however changing its focus may be.

I have the right to be cared for by those who can maintain a sense of hopefulness, however changing this might be.

I have the right to express my feelings and emotions about my approaching death in my own way.

I have the right to participate in decisions concerning my care.

I have the right to expect continuing medical and nursing attention even though "cure" goals must be changed to "comfort" goals.

I have the right not to die alone.

I have the right to be free from pain.

I have the right to have my questions answered honestly.

I have the right not to be deceived.

I have the right to have help from and for my family in accepting my death.

I have the right to die in peace and dignity.

I have the right to retain my individuality and not be judged for my decisions that may be contrary to beliefs of others.

I have the right to discuss and enlarge my religious and/or spiritual experiences, whatever these may mean to others.

I have the right to expect that the sanctity of the human body will be respected after death.

I have the right to be cared for by caring, sensitive, knowledgeable people who will attempt to understand my needs and will be able to gain some satisfaction from helping me face my death.

From Barbus AJ: The dying person's bill of rights, *Am J Nurse* 75:99, 1975.

SUMMARY

Communication is an integral part of daily life, but being able to communicate well is a skill that must be learned and refined. Remember that both your actions and words tell others about you and the imaging profession.

All patients have the right to have information about their medical condition and treatments. Spend time developing and improving your communication skills to ensure you are communicating this information in a manner appropriate for each patient's needs, life experiences, cultural background, and level of understanding. Listen empathetically, and demonstrate a caring attitude. Communication is a two-way process, and when dealing with patients, families, and other health care professionals, you must ensure that the person you are speaking with completely understands your message.

STUDY QUESTIONS

1. Diagram the communication process model and explain each of the steps.
2. Describe two problems that may occur while communicating.
3. Give two examples of nonverbal communication and describe their impact on patient communication.
4. Give one example of each of the following levels of communication:
   a. Intrapersonal
   b. Interpersonal
   c. Public
5. Describe the levels of personal space you encounter when performing a chest radiograph on a patient. Why is each level important? How should you act in each level?
6. Describe two key principles related to effective patient teaching.
7. List three possible cultural barriers and explain how each could be overcome.
8. What factors could cause an inpatient with a preexisting sensory alteration to feel a loss of self-esteem?
9. Differentiate among sensory deficit, sensory deprivation, and sensory overload, and give an example of each type of sensory alteration that is commonly found in a hospital environment.
10. Describe five communication aids and explain when and how they can be used.
11. What is the last sense lost as a person becomes unconscious?
12. Describe the behaviors typical of patients in a chemically altered state.
13. What is the Americans with Disabilities Act of 1990 and why is it important to you?
14. Specify the five stages of the grieving process. Why is each stage important?
15. Why is it important to help a dying patient remain as autonomous as possible?
16. Briefly describe the concept of hospice.

CASE STUDY

Mr. Gomez is an elderly Mexican-American patient who has come to the radiology department for an abdominal radiograph. He has been diagnosed with colon cancer and has undergone a surgical procedure that resulted in a colostomy. He speaks very little English. His wife and daughter are with him. His wife is visibly upset and uncomfortable being in the hospital. How would you explain the procedure to Mr. Gomez? Would you involve his family? In what way?

Mr. Gomez is very uncomfortable lying flat on his back and says that he just wants to be left alone to die. How would you handle this situation?

C H A P T E R

Three

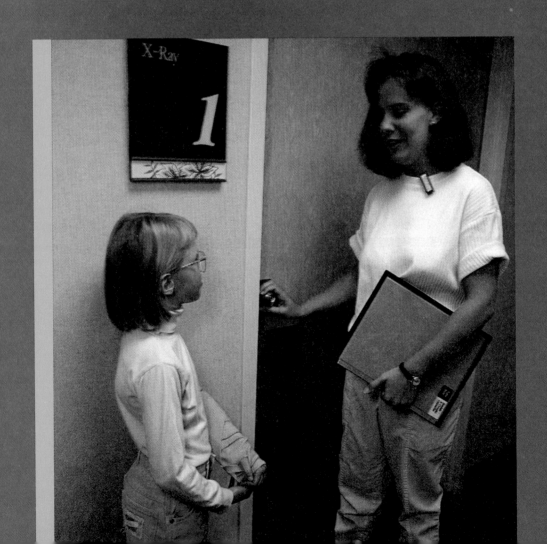

Age-Related Considerations

Key Terms

ADOLESCENT (P. 47)

AGEISM (P. 55)

DEVELOPMENT (P. 44)

GERIATRICS (P. 54)

GROWTH (P. 44)

INFANT (P. 47)

NATURE (P. 44)

NEONATE (P. 47)

NURTURE (P. 44)

PEDIATRICS (P. 47)

PRESCHOOLER (P. 47)

SCHOOL-AGE CHILD (P. 47)

TODDLER (P. 47)

Contents

Objectives

AFTER COMPLETING THIS CHAPTER, THE STUDENT WILL BE ABLE TO:

1. List the chronological stages of growth and development.
2. Differentiate between growth and development and discuss their interdependence.
3. Identify nature and nurture factors that influence growth and development.
4. Describe the key concepts relating to and techniques for communicating with infants, toddlers, preschoolers, school-age children, and adolescents.
5. Discuss physical growth characteristics for each childhood stage.
6. Discuss the different cognitive and psychosocial developmental stages during childhood, and explain how the differences affect communication with each age group.
7. Discuss the health-related concerns for neonates, infants, toddlers, school-age children, and adolescents.
8. Describe the physiologic and psychologic changes in the elderly and how these changes are important in the imaging department.

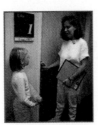

YOU WILL ENCOUNTER A VARIED PATIENT POP-
ulation while working in an imaging department.
You should therefore be familiar with factors that
influence patients' behavior and cooperation. Patient safety is always a concern, especially for elderly and very young patients. Understanding the
stages of growth and development will help you
perform safe diagnostic examinations and ensure that you use communication skills appropriate to the patient's age.

GROWTH AND DEVELOPMENT

To promote good health and deliver quality health care, you need a
basic understanding of growth and development. Human growth
and development are predictable processes that occur in an orderly
way. Growth and development are simultaneous and interdepen-
dent. They begin at conception and end at death (Table 3-1). As a
health care professional, you should be aware of the growth and developmental factors and their implications for your interactions
with patients.

People grow and develop at individual rates, but their ability to
progress through each phase of growth and development influences
their overall health. Remember that health is a relative concept
as described by the health-illness continuum (see Chapter 1).
Growth, a quantitative measurement, includes attributes such as
height, weight, skeletal size and development, and sexual age. **Development,** a qualitative measurement, involves aspects of human
behavior in response to the environment. A toddler, for example, is
more likely to cry when taken away from a parent for an examination than an adolescent.

Research shows that growth and development are influenced by
what are called *nature* and *nurture* factors. **Nature** factors include
temperament and genetics. **Nurture** factors include relationships
with family members and peers and actual life experiences. See the
box for the other basic principles of growth and development.

THE INFANT AND CHILD

The first stage of human growth and development is childhood. Because so many changes take place between infancy and adolescence,
the methods by which radiologic technologists can best communicate with children depend on the child's age and other developmental considerations.

Even though most of the necessary information about a child is

TABLE 3-1

CHRONOLOGY OF GROWTH AND DEVELOPMENT

STAGE	AGE SPAN	SIGNIFICANT BEHAVIORAL MILESTONES
Prenatal	Conception to birth	*Physical:* health and growth of fetus, maternal physical adjustments during pregnancy *Psychosocial:* maternal psychosocial adjustments during pregnancy
Neonatal	Birth to 1 month	*Physical:* exhibits infant attachment behaviors—rooting, sucking, grasping, clinging, visually fixates on objects and faces, has equality of body movements
Infancy	1 month to 1 year	*Physical:* lifts head, rolls, sits, crawls, pulls to stand, walks, grasps, rakes, transfers hand objects, uses pincer grasp *Psychosocial:* smiles, vocalizes, laughs, feeds self finger foods, says "Da-Da" and "Ma-Ma," plays peek-a-boo and pat-a-cake
Toddler	1 to 3 years	*Physical:* walks well forward and backward, stoops and recovers, climbs, runs, jumps in place, throws overhand, voluntarily releases hand, uses spoon, drinks from cup, scribbles, builds two- then four-block tower *Psychosocial:* indicates wants by behaviors other than crying, increases vocabulary, imitates, helps with household chores, points to body parts, recognizes animals, engages in solitary play
Preschool	3 to 6 years	*Physical:* rides tricycle, walks up then down stairs alternating feet, hops on one foot, tandem walks, draws circle progressing to cross and triangle, dresses with assistance then with supervision and finally alone *Psychosocial:* knows first name then age then last name, engages in parallel play progressing to interaction play, uses plurals and three-word sentences progressing to complex sentences, follows directions, counts
School age	6 to 11 years	*Physical:* skips, skates, tumbles, tandem walks backward, prints progressing to script, ties knots then bows *Psychosocial:* engages in interactive play with rules and eventually organized sports or activities, has significant peer relationships, enjoys hobbies, assumes complete responsibility for personal care
Adolescence	11 to 21 years	*Physical:* undergoes cognitive growth spurt, develops secondary sex characteristics, increases cognitive ability and formal operational thought *Psychosocial:* develops sense of identity and sex role, establishes independence, develops peer relationships with both sexes, develops life philosophy (values, beliefs), makes occupational decisions
Young and middle adult	21 to 65 years	*Physical/cognitive:* has established physical growth state and functioning, undergoes menopause, begins physical/physiologic degeneration, refines formal operational abilities *Psychosocial:* develops self-sufficiency, pursues vocation/occupation, has intense interpersonal relationships (most frequently marriage and children)
Older adult	65 years to death	*Physical:* has general slowing of physical and cognitive functioning *Psychosocial:* needs to establish highest degree of independence (self-sufficiency) physically possible by adapting environment to ability, continues interpersonal relationships, reflects on life accomplishments, events, and experiences

Modified from Potter PA, Perry AG: *Basic nursing: theory and practice,* ed 3, Mosby, 1995.

BASIC PRINCIPLES OF GROWTH AND DEVELOPMENT

1. Development is orderly and follows a set sequence.
2. Development is directional and proceeds along the following body axes:
   a. Cephalocaudal, in which growth proceeds from the head to the lower parts of the body
   b. Proximodistal, in which development proceeds from the central (proximal) areas of the body to the outer (peripheral)
   c. Differentiation, in which development proceeds from simple to complex
3. Development is complex yet predictable and occurs with a consistent pattern and chronology.
4. Development is unique to individuals and their genetic potential, and each individual tends to seek a maximal potential for development.
5. Development occurs through conflict and adaptation. Different aspects develop at different rates, creating periods of equilibrium and disequilibrium.
6. Development involves challenges for individuals in the form of certain tasks specific to age and ability.
7. Developmental tasks require practice and energy, the focus of which varies with each developmental stage and task accomplished.

Modified from Potter PA, Perry AG: *Fundamentals of nursing: concepts, process and practice*, ed 3, Mosby, 1993.

obtained from the child's parents, you should also allow older children to participate in the communication process. Children may give you information they are afraid to reveal in front of their parents, especially information about abuse. Never leave children unattended, even if they are properly immobilized.

While speaking with children, either kneel down in front of or sit beside them (Fig. 3-1). Talking with children at their eye level puts them at ease and helps them feel less vulnerable in unfamiliar surroundings. Use simple, direct language when explaining the imaging procedure. Be honest and tell the child what to expect. Children are much more willing to cooperate if you take the time to communicate with them calmly and gently. Sudden movements can frighten a child, so let the child initiate the first interpersonal contact. Children are especially sensitive to nonverbal cues such as facial expressions and signs of impatience. If you rush a child

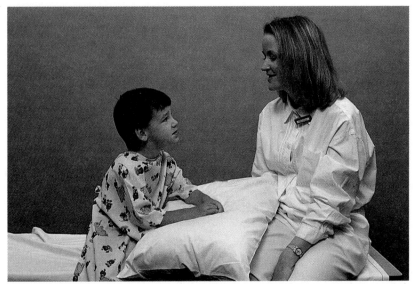

FIG. 3-1 To help put children at ease, sit beside them and explain procedures in simple terms.

through a procedure to complete an examination quickly, the child may become resistant and uncooperative. Use words the child can understand, such as comparing the x-ray tube to a camera. Avoid using technical terms that may be confusing or frightening.

Children are classified and can be better understood in terms of their age groups. Each group has its own special needs. The youngest age group is the neonate. A **neonate** is a child that is less than 28 days old. The next group classification is the infant. An **infant** is a child between the ages of 28 days and 1 year. The term **toddler** refers to a child that is 1 to 3 years old. A child 3 to 6 years of age is termed a **preschooler,** and a child 6 to 12 years old is called a **school-age child.** An **adolescent** is a child who is 13 to 18 years of age. This is a transitional period that begins at puberty and ends when the individual enters the adult world. **Pediatrics** is the branch of medicine that specializes in the care and treatment of children in all age classifications.

THE NEONATE

The average neonate weighs approximately 7 pounds and measures about 20 inches in length at birth. Neonates normally lose up to 10% of their body weight within the first few days of life and gain the weight back by the second week of life. A neonate has an average heart rate of 120 to 150 beats per minute and a respiration rate of 30 to 50 breaths per minute. Molding, or overlapping of the neonatal skull bones, is common during childbirth. Within a few weeks the bones readjust to produce a skull that appears more rounded. The sutures between the bones of the skull and the fontanels (soft spots) are palpable and clearly visible on a conventional skull radiograph.

Unless you work in a pediatric hospital, you will most likely encounter neonates in an intensive care setting. Neonates and parents normally develop an intense attachment, or bonding, within the first 28 days of the child's life. However, hospitalization of the neonate or parent may cause a delay in this bonding. Encourage parents to talk to, feed, and hold their child as much as possible during hospitalization.

Neonates have limited immune system functioning. Therefore neonatal intensive care units must strictly enforce aseptic technique practices. Individuals entering the intensive care unit (ICU) must thoroughly wash their hands. They must wear a gown and gloves before physically contacting infants. Mobile x-ray and ultrasound units must be cleaned before they are taken into the ICU. When performing a radiographic procedure on a neonate or entering the ICU, clean the cassette. The cassette must also be covered to prevent direct contact with the child.

THE INFANT

Infants develop rapidly during the first year of life. They develop cognitively, physically, and psychosocially. Infants normally triple their birth weight and greatly increase their mobility by their first birthday.

Carefully immobilize infants when performing diagnostic procedures. Immobilization devices such as a Pig-o-stat (Fig. 3-2) and papoose board should be used to obtain the necessary radiographs and ensure patient safety. Infants should never be left unattended in the department.

Vision, hearing, and verbal ability also develop rapidly during the first year. The infant progresses from crying, cooing, and laughing to imitating sounds and comprehending simple commands. By 8 months of age, infants respond differently to strangers than they do to familiar people, and they look to their parents for support and comfort. Take time to hold and comfort infants by talking to them before proceeding with examinations. Consider having parents come into the examination room during positioning to decrease childrens' anxiety about being separated from their parents.

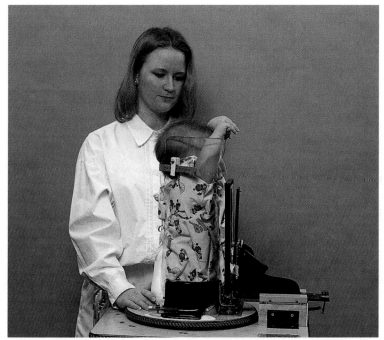

FIG. 3-2 A Pig-o-stat may be used to immobilize an infant.

THE TODDLER

Toddlers are more independent than infants and they need control of situations. Children between the ages of 1 and 3 years often throw temper tantrums and exhibit negative behavior. Because they are seldom in control of a hospital situation, they may be difficult to handle. Put children at ease by allowing them to hold a security item such as a favorite blanket or toy, or give them a small toy yourself to help develop rapport. During this stage of life, toddlers develop memories and begin to understand cause and effect.

Verbal skills continue to develop rapidly. An 18-month old can possess a vocabulary of approximately 10 words, whereas a 2-year old's vocabulary consists of about 300 words. Most children talk constantly by the age of 3 years. Take the time to establish rapport with toddlers. Acquaint them with the radiographic equipment, and explain the procedure in terms they can understand. Like infants, toddlers must be restrained during imaging procedures to prevent motion blurring. This is most easily accomplished using a sheet to

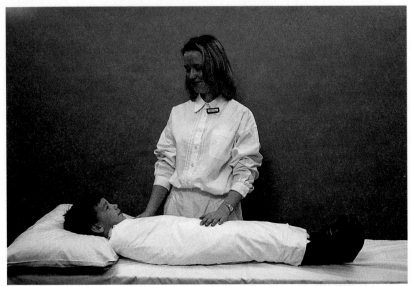

FIG. 3-3 A sheet may be used "mummy style" to immobilize a toddler.

form a "mummy" restraint (Fig. 3-3). Talk to the toddler throughout the procedure, and explain each step in understandable terms. Toddlers should never be left unattended in a radiology department.

THE PRESCHOOLER

During the preschool years, physical development begins to slow. The heart rate stabilizes at about 90 beats per minute, and the respiration rate slows to about 24 breaths per minute. Weight gain also slows during these years. The average 5-year old weighs approximately 45 pounds. An average preschooler grows about an inch taller per year. Muscle coordination improves during this stage, and children learn to walk more easily, run, navigate stairs, and hop.

Cognitive and psychosocial skills develop rapidly from 3 to 6 years of age. Problem-solving abilities develop, although the child's knowledge of the world is primarily linked to concrete experiences. Preschoolers' verbal skills continue to improve; the average 5-year old uses more than 2000 words. At this stage of development, most children can name their body parts and identify bodily sensations. Most preschool children can link events that are related in time and space. They can also wash, dress, and feed themselves quite independently.

Although preschool-aged children continue to rely on their parents for security, they begin to initiate contact with other adults and children. Preschoolers tend to be less afraid of strangers, so they may ask you a multitude of questions. Listen to what children ask you, and answer the questions honestly, using language appropriate for a preschooler. Most preschoolers will cooperate with you if they trust you.

Remember that because preschool-age children often cannot distinguish between fantasy and reality, they may be unnecessarily frightened in certain situations. For instance, you may explain to children you are restraining them in a sheet for a procedure, but preschoolers may believe they are being restrained because they are crying. As with all children, preschoolers should never be left unattended in the department, even when immobilized.

THE SCHOOL-AGE CHILD

School-age children range in age from 6 to 12 years and have usually begun formal schooling. Their educational experience influences their growth and development and expands their perceptions of the world. Children in this stage of life begin to understand and follow rules, analyze situations, make decisions, accept responsibility for their actions, and learn from life experiences.

School-age children grow steadily, gaining about 1 to 2 inches in height and approximately 3 to 6 lb per year. Females generally undergo prepubertal physical changes between the ages of 9 and 12, whereas males undergo these changes primarily in adolescence. Cardiovascular function stabilizes during this growth phase; the heart reaches adult size by age 12. The average heart beats 65 to 90 times per minute, and the average respiration rate is 16 to 18 breaths per minute. Muscle strength and large and fine motor skills dramatically improve during this period.

Skeletal changes also occur during the school-age stage of life. The bones of the trunk and extremities begin to ossify and epiphyseal growth plates are clearly visible on bone radiographs. The frontal sinuses develop at 8 to 9 years of age, and by the age of 10, most of the primary teeth have erupted and replaced the deciduous teeth. As skeletal growth progresses, the child stands more erect. This makes the detection of an abnormal curvature of the spine such as scoliosis more apparent. In addition, school-age children often undergo examinations to detect or diagnose visual or auditory abnormalities.

School-age children can understand and communicate with the world. They can think abstractly and relate past, present, and future events. At this stage, they progress from using concrete thinking to using inductive logic. Because they are more socialized than they were at earlier stages, they are able to consider the views of others. Language skills continue to develop during this period. As their vocabulary increases, school-age children begin to understand that words have relative rather than absolute meaning and that words may have more than one definition.

Because accidents and injuries are a major health problem for children at this stage, you will often see school-age children in the emergency department. The leading causes of death for school-age children are motor vehicle and recreational activity accidents. In this stage many children develop a fear of illness, injury, and death. Because they are inquisitive, they may ask many health-related questions. Be open and honest with them and explain procedures in a language they can understand. This will help diminish their fears by providing them with an informed understanding of the situation.

THE ADOLESCENT

During the stage of life from 13 to 18 years of age, the child makes the transition into adulthood. Physical, cognitive, and psychosocial changes force adolescents to develop coping mechanisms for adapting to new situations. Adolescents are establishing an identity and making major life decisions. This time period is one of great stress for both adolescents and their parents.

Sexual maturation occurs during adolescence, as does an increased skeletal and muscular growth rate. Height and weight increase significantly during this pubertal growth spurt, and adolescents often become very sensitive about these physical changes. These patients are often very modest, so allow them to put on the examination gown in a private setting, and offer them a robe.

Adolescents not only have the cognitive ability to think logically but can also reason abstractly. They can use deductive reasoning and understand abstract hypothetical situations. Language development is nearly complete at this age, but communication skills are still developing. Adolescents often express their feelings to and share knowledge with their parents and peers. The communication skills they develop at this stage will be used throughout adulthood. Always treat adolescents as adults while explaining an imaging procedure.

During this stage, young people begin to judge themselves against internalized ideals. They decide which rules to apply to themselves. Adolescents need to make choices and experience the consequences of their actions. Independence is crucial to achieving a personal identity.

TECHNIQUES FOR COMMUNICATING WITH CHILDREN

INFANTS

Infants communicate primarily nonverbally (cooing, smiling, and crying) and seek comfort. Avoid loud, harsh sounds and sudden movements. Gentle, close physical contact helps infants to become quiet. Keep the patients in view while holding and interacting with infants.

TODDLERS OR PRESCHOOLERS

Toddlers communicate verbally and nonverbally. They are egocentric with all activities focused on the self. Speech and thought processes are concrete. Focus discussion on the childrens' personal needs and concerns. Tell toddlers specifically what to do and how they will feel. Allow them to explore the environment (by handling a stethoscope or playing with a tongue blade). Use simple, short sentences, familiar words, and concrete explanations. Avoid ambiguous phrases toddlers cannot interpret, such as: "The shot will just feel like a bee sting", or "Take this medicine for your your tummy ache."

SCHOOL-AGE CHILDREN

The speech of school-age children is primarily verbal. They seek explanations about the world and are interested in functional aspects of objects and events. These children are concerned about body integrity. Give simple explanations. Demonstrate how equipment works. Allow children to manipulate equipment (e.g., hold a percussion hammer or wear a stethoscope). Allow children to express fears or concerns.

ADOLESCENTS

Adolescents think more abstractly, fluctuate between childish and adult thinking behavior, and like talking with adults outside of the family. Avoid imposing values or judgments. Allow the adolescents time to talk. Be attentive and avoid interrupting them or showing gestures of disapproval. Avoid embarrassing questions or the impulse to give advice. Adolescents frequently use a language of their own, so clarify their terms, as well as your own.

Modified from Potter PA, Perry AG: *Basic nursing: theory and practice*, ed 3, Mosby, 1995.

As with school-age children the leading cause of injury and death during the adolescent years is accidents that are primarily caused by motor vehicles. Motor vehicle accidents may be associated with alcohol, drug abuse, or depression. Sexually transmitted diseases are the most common communicable illness in this age group, so health education should provide accurate information about preventing pregnancy and sexually transmitted diseases. The box describes communication techniques that can be used with children at different developmental stages.

THE OLDER ADULT

Aging is inevitable, regardless of gender, socioeconomic status, or cultural background. The older adult is at the last stage of growth and development. Over the past decade the medical needs of older people have received greater emphasis than they have in the past. The branch of medicine that deals with the physiologic and psychologic changes of the elderly and diagnoses and treats their diseases is called **geriatrics.**

The field of geriatrics has expanded as the average age of the U.S. population has grown increasingly older. This demographic shift is partly connected to a decline in the birth rate and to an aging "baby boom" generation. Technologic advances have also contributed to increased longevity. In addition to these factors, there has been increased attention to improving the quality of life for older adults both medically and socially. Examples include the establishment of extended care facilities and independent living arrangements in retirement communities.

PHYSIOLOGIC CONSIDERATIONS

Physical and cognitive functioning generally slows as the human body ages. Bones tend to lose calcium, body tissues lose elasticity, and muscle strength diminishes. These physiologic changes are responsible for many of the health care problems of the elderly.

Older adults have a greater risk of developing respiratory problems such as pulmonary congestion and pneumonia. Many elderly patients are hypertensive due to a lack of tissue elasticity. Poor blood circulation increases older adults' sensitivity to temperature changes and pain and in some cases may lead to vertigo and fainting. The elderly are also more prone to coronary artery disease, strokes, malignant neoplasms, and arthritis.

Most injuries to older patients involve falls, burns, and motor vehicle accidents. Elderly patients are the primary consumers of prescription drugs; the side effects of medication increase the risk of injury resulting from falls. The older adult may find it difficult to physically tolerate the position changes necessary to obtain quality diagnostic images. Be aware of these physiologic difficulties to ensure quality patient care and prevent injury.

Approximately 75% of older adults have at least one chronic health problem, so you are likely to interact daily with geriatric patients in your imaging department. Elderly patients may become disoriented because the imaging department environment is unfamiliar. Be sure to orient patients to their surroundings. Tell them they are in the x-ray department and that you will stay with them during the procedure. Be sure to explain to patients the reason they are having the procedure.

Physiologic changes within the body may lead to diminished hearing and vision; communicate clearly with older adults, and consider their special needs (Fig. 3-4). Do not yell. Instead, speak in a normal tone close to the patient's ear. Speak slowly and articulate

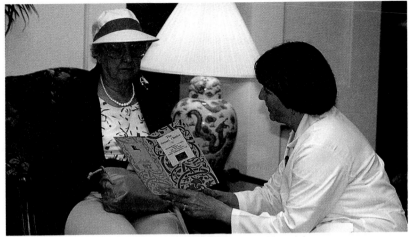

FIG. 3-4 Communicate clearly to older adults.

clearly. To communicate with a hearing-impaired patient who can read lips, position yourself so that the patient can see your lips move. When possible, reduce background noise to eliminate distractions. Always introduce yourself to older adults when you enter their hospital rooms to perform bedside examinations.

PSYCHOLOGIC CONSIDERATIONS

Even though aging is inevitable, older adults often find it difficult to accept that they are growing older. Many stereotypes and myths exist about the elderly. This can lead to a bias against the elderly, which is a prejudice referred to as **ageism.**

People who are ageists believe that the elderly lack understanding, have poor memories, are rigid, spend most of their time drowsing, and are unpleasant to others. Stereotypes and myths like these have no place in the health care field. Each elderly person is an individual. In fact, most older adults are physically and socially active. Only 5% of people older than 65 require nursing home or institutional care. However, changes in the aged person's lifestyle, such as losing a spouse or having a decreased activity level, may result in special psychologic needs.

Health care professionals should understand and empathize with people who are experiencing the aging process. Older adults have had to adjust to many physical changes brought about by age. The elderly possess a wealth of knowledge and, because of their individual life experiences, often have a unique perspective on social, economic, and technologic developments and issues.

Many older adults must adjust to living on fixed incomes. In our culture, retirement sometimes results in passivity and seclusion; thus retirement from full-time employment can lead to unique psychosocial stresses. Retirement may lead to changing roles within a marriage or family or to social isolation. Many older adults choose to participate in volunteer activities to maintain an active social life. Continued socialization and a sufficient income are important factors that affect the quality of life of older adults.

Many older adults have suffered through the death of a spouse, of friends, and sometimes even of their children. These losses are very difficult to resolve, and normal grieving may take many months. The death of a loved one also diminishes the breadth of the older adult's social circle.

Physical limitations and physiologic changes may require a change in the older adult's living arrangements, such as moving to a retirement community, into an extended care facility, or in with adult children. These changes may result in redefined relationships between older parents and their adult children, especially if the changes involve a role reversal in which the parent becomes dependent on the child. This adds psychosocial stress for older adults and may lead to feelings of guilt or low self-esteem.

Be aware of the psychologic effects of aging so that you can better communicate with and meet the needs of this population. Older adults have much to offer our society and should not be stereotyped. Acknowledge the limitations of aging, but respect the wisdom of the aged.

SUMMARY

Every patient is unique and should be treated as an individual. Understanding the most appropriate means of communicating with patients will increase their cooperation with you in the imaging department. As you become more experienced in your profession, you will find that you use the principles of growth and development more as you strive to meet the needs of patients in all age groups.

1. Differentiate between growth and development.
2. Differentiate between nature and nurture factors that affect growth and development.
3. Describe at least four of the seven basic principles of growth and development.
4. Why is aseptic technique important in a neonatal intensive care area? In what way does this affect the radiologic technologist?
5. Name two types of pediatric immobilization devices, and explain how and why each is used.
6. Describe the appropriate verbal communication techniques for explaining an imaging procedure to the following age groups:
   a. Toddlers
   b. Preschoolers
   c. School-age children
7. What physical changes take place during the school-age and adolescent years that are important to consider when performing an imaging procedure on these patients?
8. List two common health problems of the elderly, and explain why these may be important in the imaging department.
9. Identify two common myths about older adults.
10. Explain how the various psychologic changes and stresses experienced by a geriatric patient may affect communication with them in the imaging department.

Four

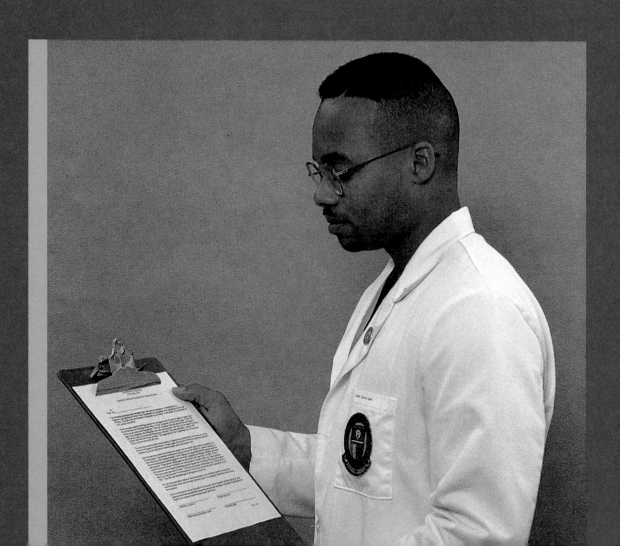

Medical Ethics and Legalities

Key Terms

Contents

Objectives

AFTER COMPLETING THIS CHAPTER, THE STUDENT WILL BE ABLE TO:

1. Compare and discuss moral, ethical, and legal issues relevant to the field of health care.
2. Explain the importance of the ARRT Code of Ethics, including the technologist's responsibility and accountability to patients and to their field.
3. Demonstrate the way critical thinking skills are used to resolve ethical dilemmas.
4. Explain the importance of the Patient's Bill of Rights.
5. Describe the ways "standard of care" and "scope of practice" relate to radiologic technology.

6. Differentiate between criminal and civil law and describe the various civil law violations relevant to health care professionals.
7. List the criteria necessary to obtain a valid informed consent.
8. Discuss legal concepts related to professional practice.

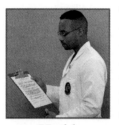 THE VALUES AND CULTURAL DIFFERENCES discussed in Chapter 2 are directly related to the ethical and legal aspects of radiologic technology discussed in this chapter. Just as patients enter the health care system with their own values, health care providers also have personal values, and these may influence decisions about patient care. Health care professionals should protect human rights using established professional standards. Staying objective in all situations that involve personal values and patient rights is critical if you are going to effectively respond to patients' needs knowledgeably and with discipline.

In any health care setting the health care provider, the patient, and society as a whole may have conflicting values. Differences in values can lead to ethical dilemmas. For instance, although medical technologic advances have made it possible to keep terminally ill patients alive for long periods, the care of these patients often presents ethical dilemmas. When should and should not life-sustaining procedures be performed? At what point do you stop performing diagnostic procedures when you know they will not actually affect a patient's ultimate outcome?

VALUES AND ETHICS

Values may be defined as the worth or importance a person places on a reality or an idea. In other words, values are a person's established ideals of life. Personal values are influenced by needs and relationships with others as well as culture and society. Values are often wrapped up in powerful emotions and govern the way an individual acts or reacts in a given situation.

The term *ethics* comes from the Greek word *ethos* meaning "custom." Ethics may be defined as a system of standards defining what is right and wrong. Ethical principles are often associated with professional rules or actions professionals should take in given situations.

An ethical dilemma occurs when two different ethical systems conflict and there is no obvious right or wrong resolution. Ethical dilemmas may result when your **ethics** and a patient's ethics conflict or when your professional duty to a patient and a health care facility conflict. Resolving these conflicts requires a knowledge of moral, ethical, and legal standards. **Moral values** are personal convictions about absolute rights and wrongs. For example, many people have strong personal convictions about the morality of euthanasia. However, when confronted with an issue like this, you must comply with the ethical and legal standards of a health care professional. A moral issue only becomes an ethical issue when there is no clear application of the universal principles of right and wrong. Resolving an ethical issue may require an individual to choose between solutions that are all fairly pleasant, but it also may require choosing between options that are all undesirable.

Ethical and legal standards are often closely related. Ethical standards govern proper professional conduct, which includes professional decisions and actions. An ethical issue, for example, could arise when considering whether to extend the life of a terminally ill, comatose patient. Ethical arguments could be made for and against extending this patient's life. In addition, the **legal rights** of the individuals involved would have to be considered. Legal rights are the privileges entitled to individuals within the limits of the law.

In addition, you need to realize that morality and legality may not always agree. You may personally find an individual's actions morally wrong even if they are legal, or you may believe certain actions are morally acceptable although they are illegal. In addition, although your personal morals and ethics may not agree with a patient's beliefs, you should abide by the ethical standards set by your profession when resolving conflicts.

PROFESSIONAL ETHICS

Most ethical dilemmas arise in situations that require difficult decisions regarding patient care. In some cases, ethical dilemmas force you to choose between options that are equally unsatisfactory. **Professional ethics** are the principles or standards that define right and wrong within a profession. These principles can help you make the most appropriate decisions in ambiguous situations.

The **American Registry of Radiologic Technologists' (ARRT) code of ethics** delineates the profession's high ideals of conduct (box). The code assures the public that radiologic technologists will not exploit their positions as health care professionals. Each registered technologist must uphold these standards.

The ARRT Code of Ethics also helps a radiologic technologist determine proper conduct in specific situations. The principles of conduct are based on respecting self-determination and autonomy, doing good and avoiding harm (nonmaleficence), being honest, keeping promises, and maintaining confidentiality (respecting privileged information). To uphold the code, you must be responsible and accountable for your actions.

THE AMERICAN REGISTRY OF RADIOLOGIC TECHNOLOGISTS CODE OF ETHICS

This Code shall serve as a guide by which Radiologic Technologists may evaluate their professional conduct as it relates to patients, colleagues, other members of the medical care team, health care consumers and employers. The Code is intended to assist radiologic technologists in maintaining a high level of ethical conduct.

1. The Radiologic Technologist conducts himself/herself in a professional manner, responds to patient needs and supports colleagues and associates in providing quality patient care.

2. The Radiologic Technologist acts to advance the principal objective of the profession to provide services to humanity with full respect for the dignity of mankind.

3. The Radiologic Technologist delivers patient care and service unrestricted by the concerns of personal attributes or the nature of the disease or illness, and without discrimination regardless of sex, race, creed, religion, or socioeconomic status.

4. The Radiologic Technologist practices technology founded upon theoretical knowledge and concepts, utilizes equipment and accessories consistent with the purposes for which they have been designed, and employs procedures and techniques appropriately.

5. The Radiologic Technologist assesses situations, exercises care, discretion and judgment, assumes responsibility for professional decisions, and acts in the best interest of the patient.

6. The Radiologic Technologist acts as an agent through observation and communication to obtain pertinent information for the physician to aid in the diagnosis and treatment management of the patient, and recognizes that interpretation and diagnosis are outside the scope of practice for the profession.

7. The Radiologic Technologist utilizes equipment and accessories, employs techniques and procedures, performs services in accordance with an accepted standard of practice, and demonstrates expertise in limiting the radiation exposure to the patient, self, and other members of the health care team.

8. The Radiologic Technologist practices ethical conduct appropriate to the profession and protects the patient's right to quality radiologic technology care.

9. The Radiologic Technologist respects confidences entrusted in the course of professional practice, respects the patient's right to privacy, and reveals confidential information only as required by law or to protect the welfare of the individual or the community.

10. The Radiologic Technologist continually strives to improve knowledge and skills by participating in educational and professional activities, sharing knowledge with colleagues and investigating new and innovative aspects of professional practice. One means available to improve knowledge and skill is through professional continuing education.

From The American Registry of Radiologic Technologists, 1993, The Registry.

Radiologic technologists have a **responsibility** to perform all duties ethically, which helps in gaining credibility and earning the trust of patients, other health care professionals, and the general public.

A responsible radiologic technologist performs radiographic examinations safely and maintains the dignity, confidentiality, and physical and psychologic safety of each patient. Proper patient positioning, production of high quality radiographs, and proper administration of medications are essential components of a responsible practice. Being informed and clinically competent are necessary to perform responsibly within the ethical guidelines of the profession.

Radiologic technology professionals must have an **accountability** to their actions, themselves, patients, their employers, and society in general. Self-accountability includes reporting any personal actions that endanger a patient, making judgments based on factual information, and maintaining your competence in current radiologic technology techniques.

Being accountabile to patients means ensuring patient safety while conducting radiologic procedures. Producing quality images necessary for accurate diagnoses and giving patients and their families accurate information about procedures are also aspects of being accountable to patients. Accountability to your employer requires honesty, appropriate use of supplies, and adherence to institutional policies and procedures. Accountability to society means you must care for every patient, regardless of age, gender, race, creed, socioeconomic status, disabilities, or health problems. In addition, to ensure professional excellence, you must adhere to the ethics of practice, maintain self-discipline, and report unethical behavior.

SKILLS FOR RESOLVING ETHICAL PROBLEMS

Critical thinking skills are important when resolving ethical problems. Evaluate problems to ensure they are ethical problems and not communication or legal problems. Most ethical dilemmas are a result of conflicting principles that lead to equally undesirable options for resolutions. For instance, determining whether it is necessary to perform a barium enema examination on an 80-year-old patient who has been diagnosed with an advanced stage of breast cancer is a difficult situation. There is no "right" or "wrong" decision and the determination cannot be made by scientific data alone. The resolution should be approached systematically and all available options considered.

CRITICAL THINKING SKILLS

Although no two ethical dilemmas are the same, you should always use a systematic decision-making process when resolving problems. Consider the ethical principles and values related to the specific situation. A systematic approach should include the following key steps:

1. List everyone involved in the decision-making process. Identify their perceptions of the problems and possible solutions.
2. Presume everyone involved in the decision-making process is considering the well-being of the patient.
3. Gather relevant and factual information.
4. Clarify the ethical issues involved. Everyone involved should list possible resolutions.
5. Determine the strengths of each possible resolution by listing the positive attributes of each. Compare and rank each resolution.
6. Use the best resolution.

True ethical problems have no right and wrong answers. Focus on the patient's outcome and quality of life. Ethical decisions should not be made solely by one professional because the decision may be rejected. Resolutions must incorporate the collective decisions of everyone involved—the health care workers, the patient, the patient's family members, and any significant others. A systematic approach that includes everyone involved helps resolve ethical issues consistently, objectively, and professionally.

LEGAL CONSIDERATIONS

Laws enable our society to handle disputes systematically and fairly. Laws are the rules and regulations that are necessary to govern a society, and many of them vary in different states.

Be aware of specific state statutes that affect your profession. For example, many states require professionals practicing radiography, nuclear medicine technology, or radiation oncology to be licensed. State licensing acts generally delineate the professional's **scope of practice,** in addition to educational requirements and legal practice guidelines necessary to ensure public safety. Licensure allows only individuals who have demonstrated they are skilled in and knowledgeable about the radiologic sciences to perform radiologic procedures.

PATIENT RIGHTS

Society emphasizes patient and consumer rights. Health care practitioners must understand their legal obligations and responsibilities to patients. The American Hospital Association has developed the Patient's Bill of Rights (box). Although this is not a legal document because it is not a law, it helps set guidelines for patient care throughout the country.

STANDARDS OF CARE

Laws establish standards of care for health care professionals. Other professions also have detailed explicit standards of care, such as the Nursing Practice Act for nursing. Radiologic technology's standards are defined by the American Society of Radiologic Technologists in their "scope of care" (box). The scope of care establishes the whats, hows, and whys of radiologic technology practice. These standards are continually updated to reflect technologic advances in the profession. The scope of care describes the technologist's general responsibilities, accountabilities, and guidelines by which to practice.

Standards of care are important for both legal and ethical reasons. Health care professionals who do not follow accepted standards of care risk becoming involved in legal disputes.

BASIC LEGAL CONCEPTS

There are two types of law: criminal and civil. **Criminal law** deals with individuals who threaten society. Individuals accused of criminal offenses are arrested and prosecuted in the criminal justice system.

Crimes are categorized as either felonies or misdemeanors. A felony is a serious crime and may lead to a heavy fine, imprisonment, or the death penalty. The penalties for misdemeanors, which are less serious crimes, are usually fines or less than a year of imprisonment. Criminal law cases rarely play a part in health care unless health care professionals are not practicing within accepted standards of care.

Civil law is based on precedents and principles; it does not have written codes with penalties. Violations are prosecuted in civil court. A civil wrong committed against an individual or an individual's property is called a **tort.** An individual who sues another individual or institution is claiming a tort has taken place. Torts may involve intentional or unintentional actions. An intentional tort is willfully violating another's rights. For instance, forcing a patient to undergo a radiologic procedure when the patient has refused treatment is an intentional tort. Performing below the normal standard of care, such as forgetting to check a patient's identification band

YOUR RIGHTS AS A HOSPITAL PATIENT

We consider you a partner in your hospital care. When you are well-informed, participate in treatment decisions, and communicate openly with your doctor and other health professionals, you help make your care as effective as possible. This hospital encourages respect for the personal preferences and values of each individual.

While you are a patient in the hospital, your rights include the following:

- You have the right to considerate and respectful care.
- You have the right to be well-informed about your illness, possible treatments, and likely outcome and to discuss this information with your doctor. You have the right to know the names and roles of people treating you.
- You have the right to consent to or refuse a treatment, as permitted by law, throughout your hospital stay. If you refuse a recommended treatment, you will receive other needed and available care.
- You have the right to have an advance directive, such as a living will or health care proxy. These documents express your choices about your future care or name someone to decide if you cannot speak for yourself. If you have a written advance directive, you should provide a copy to the hospital, your family, and your doctor.
- You have the right to privacy. The hospital, your doctor, and others caring for you will protect your privacy as much as possible.
- You have the right to expect that treatment records are confidential unless you have given permission to release information or reporting is required or permitted by law. When the hospital releases records to others, such as insurers, it emphasizes that the records are confidential.
- You have the right to review your medical records and to have the information explained, except when restricted by law.
- You have the right to expect that the hospital will give you necessary health services to the best of its ability. Treatment, referral, or transfer may be recommended. If transfer is recommended or requested, you will be informed of risks, benefits, and alternatives. You will not be transferred until the other institution agrees to accept you.
- You have the right to know if this hospital has relationships with outside parties that may influence your treatment and care. These relationships may be with educational institutions, other health care providers, or insurers.
- You have the right to consent or decline to take part in research affecting your care. If you choose not to take part, you will receive the most effective care the hospital otherwise provides.
- You have the right to be told of realistic care alternatives when hospital care is no longer appropriate.
- You have the right to know about hospital rules that affect you and your treatment and about charges and payment methods. You have the right to know about hospital resources, such as patient representatives or ethics committees, that can help you resolve problems and questions about your hospital stay and care.

You have responsibilities as a patient. You are responsible for providing information about your health, including past illnesses, hospital stays, and use of medicine. You are responsible for asking questions when you do not understand information or instructions. If you believe you can't follow through with your treatment, you are responsible for telling your doctor.

This hospital works to provide care efficiently and fairly to all patients and the community. You and your visitors are responsible for being considerate of the needs of other patients, staff, and the hospital. You are responsible for providing information for insurance and for working with the hospital to arrange payment, when needed.

Your health depends not just on your hospital care but, in the long term, on the decisions you make in your daily life. You are responsible for recognizing the effect of life-style on your personal health.

A hospital serves many purposes. Hospitals work to improve people's health; treat people with injury and disease; educate doctors, health professionals, patients, and community members; and improve understanding of health and disease. In carrying out these activities, this institution works to respect your values and dignity.

From American Hospital Association, 1992, The Association.

THE SCOPE OF PRACTICE

RADIOGRAPHER—RT(R)(ARRT)

1. Completion of a formal program of study accredited by the Committee on Allied Health Education and Accreditation of the American Medical Association in collaboration with the American Society of Radiologic Technologists and the American College of Radiology, which sponsor the Joint Review Committee on Education in Radiologic Technology.
   OR
   Completion of didactic and clinical experience acceptable to the American Registry of Radiologic Technologists.
   AND
2. Certification by the American Registry of Radiologic Technologists.

The art and science of radiography that the radiographer achieve a specific level of knowledge and skill. The radiographer must possess and demonstrate knowledge of and competency in, but not limited to, the following areas:

HUMAN STRUCTURE AND FUNCTION—including general anatomy, cross-sectional anatomy and anatomic relationships, organ and organ system functions and relationships in order to perform accurate radiographic examinations.

MEDICAL ETHICS—including ethical and legal considerations that impact upon practice.

MEDICAL TERMINOLOGY—including knowledge of disease and abnormalities to allow the radiologic technologist to effectively communicate in the performance of radiographic procedures.

PATHOLOGY—including knowledge of disease and abnormalities that influence performance of radiographic procedures.

PATIENT CARE—including attention and concern for the physical and psychological needs of the patient. Additionally, the technologist identifies the accurate assessment of life-threatening conditions and exercises independent judgment to implement basic life support procedures.

POSITIONING—including proper beam-part-image receptor alignment with respect to source of radiation selected imaging modality, and area to be examined.

PRINCIPLES OF RADIOGRAPHIC EXPOSURE—including appropriate selection of all technical factors and equipment to produce a quality diagnostic radiograph.

QUALITY ASSURANCE—including darkroom chemistry and processing procedures, sensitometry characteristics, preventive maintenance, and knowledge of equipment.

RADIATION PHYSICS—including atomic structure, beam quality, radiation interactions, and the functions and operations of various generator components.

RADIATION PROTECTION—including the use of beam restrictive devices, patient shielding techniques, proper screen-film combinations, accurate assessment and implementation of appropriate exposure factors as well as a working understanding of applicable governmental regulations. The primary utilization of this knowledge to minimize radiation to the patient, the practitioner, and others.

RADIOBIOLOGY—including understanding of beam formation and radiation interaction with matter as it relates to genetic and somatic effects. The necessity for this knowledge and its application is to reduce possible genetic damage to future generations resulting from unnecessary radiation exposure.

SPECIAL TECHNIQUES—including all vascular and neurological radiographic procedures, computed tomography, magnetic resonance, mammography, and interventional radiography.

The practice of radiography is stated as the performance, for compensation or personal profit, of service including, but not limited to:

- Radiographic examinations, upon the order of a physician, of all body parts for diagnostic interpretation by a physician.
- Optimal patient care utilizing established and accepted techniques.
- Supervision of other practitioners where applicable.
- Supervision and instruction of students where applicable.
- Evaluation of the above functions and recommendations for improvement.

From The American Society of Radiologic Technologists, The Society.

before a radiologic procedure, is negligence. This is an example of an unintentional tort.

The purpose of a civil case is generally to compensate the client who brought suit rather than to punish the person accused of the tort. In contrast, the purpose of a criminal suit is generally to punish the criminal. Common health care torts include negligence or malpractice, assault, battery, invasion of privacy, false imprisonment, and defamation of character.

NEGLIGENCE AND MALPRACTICE

Negligence occurs when a health care professional provides substandard care. A negligent health care professional does not provide care as competently as a prudent practitioner does under the same circumstances.

Although negligence is generally a result of thoughtlessness or inattention to detail, incompetence that harms a patient is also negligence. Examples of negligent conduct include failing to prevent a patient fall that results in injury and injecting a patient with an incorrect type or amount of contrast material.

Malpractice can be a result of professional misconduct or an unreasonable incompetence or lack of skills. In a malpractice lawsuit the burden of proof is on the patient. This means that the patient must establish that the four following statements are true:

1. The radiologic technologist owed a duty to the patient.
2. The radiologic technologist did not carry out this duty.
3. The patient was injured.
4. The patient's injury was a result of radiologic technologist's failure to carry out the duty.

The best way to avoid a malpractice lawsuit is to practice competently. Stay within your scope of care, meet all standards of care, and develop rapport with each patient. Patients must understand procedures and should be well-informed about risks associated with specific examinations or treatments (Fig. 4-1).

ASSAULT AND BATTERY

Assault is willfully attempting or threatening to harm someone. An assault does not have to involve physical contact. An assault can be subtle; coercing patients into undergoing radiologic procedures against their will could be considered assault. Assault can also be as obvious as actually threatening another person. For instance, telling children they will never see their parents again if they do not hold still for a radiograph is assault.

Battery is intentionally touching another individual without consent. The individual does not have to be injured to claim battery.

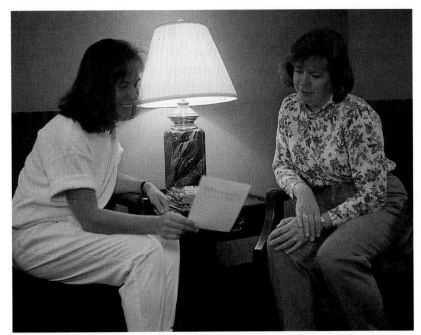

FIG. 4-1 Carefully explain the procedure to the patient before beginning the examination.

For example, performing a radiologic procedure on a patient who has refused treatment is battery.

Touching patients is a necessary part of performing a radiologic procedure. Although patient consent for routine procedures is given on admission to the hospital, before beginning to position patients, you should obtain permission from them for specific procedures. Informed consent and implied consent are important when interacting with patients in the imaging department.

Written, informed consent is not necessary for all procedures. Consent may be implied by the patient's actions and acceptance of hospital care. For instance, if a patient follows your preparation directions for a chest x-ray and you have explained the procedure, the patient has implied that it is acceptable for you to perform the procedure.

INVASION OF PRIVACY

All patients are entitled to confidential health care. Medical records, including the patient histories and all other information, are considered privileged and confidential information. Look at records only when they are pertinent for a procedure you are performing.

For instance, it is not necessary to know a patient's HIV status unless it is relevant to the radiologic examination being performed.

Diagnostic images and radiology film records are considered part of the medical record. They must be handled confidentially like a patient's chart. Medical information should only be shared with individuals who are involved in the patient's care and must know for treatment purposes.

An **invasion of privacy** can be as obvious as releasing medical information to the press or as subtle as discussing a patient's condition with a co-worker in a public place (like an elevator). Maintain confidentiality and ensure the privacy of each patient.

FALSE IMPRISONMENT

False imprisonment issues may arise in imaging departments that are using restraints. Physical restraints are devices used to immobilize patients. Drugs may also be considered a form of restraint when presented by a physician to decrease patient activity in extreme cases. Patients restrained against their will could have a false imprisonment claim.

Restraints can be used to reduce the risk of patient falls or to prevent confused or combative patients from removing their endotracheal tubes, nasogastric tubes, indwelling urinary catheters, intravenous lines, and so on. Patients should never be restrained, however, for the convenience of the staff. Technologists should only restrain or immobilize a patient when it is absolutely necessary for the patient's safety. You must follow your institution's specific guidelines, policies, and procedures when using restraints. Patients must be informed of the reasons they are being restrained. You must obtain parental or guardian consent when restraining pediatric patients (Fig. 4-2) or patients in an altered state of consciousness (such as confused and intoxicated patients) who are unable to comprehend their situation.

DEFAMATION OF CHARACTER

Defamation of character occurs when an individual's reputation is harmed. Defamation through spoken communication is called *slander*, and defamation through written communication is called *libel*. Telling someone a co-worker is incompetent could be considered slander. Making intentionally damaging statements or relaying false information about another person is also slander. Writing a comment in a medical record regarding someone's incompetence could be considered libel.

Disclosing confidential information about patients to their employers and therefore causing them to lose their jobs or suffer in any

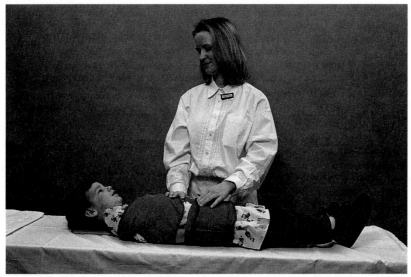

FIG. 4-2 You must obtain parental permission to restrain pediatric patients for radiologic procedures.

way is also considered defamation of character. The disclosure of confidential information to the press resulting in public ridicule, scorn, or contempt of an individual is also considered defamation of character.

INFORMED CONSENT

When patients agree to particular procedures or treatments after receiving all necessary facts, the agreement is called an **informed consent.** Before you perform any invasive, interventional, or potentially hazardous procedures such as angiograms, patients must sign a consent form (Fig. 4-3).

Informed consent is valid when the following conditions are met:

1. The consenting individual is a legal adult who is mentally and physically competent.
2. Consent is given voluntarily.
3. The consenting individual understands the procedure, its risks, and its benefits.
4. The consenting individual's right to have all questions answered satisfactorily has been respected.

If a patient is not a legal adult, a parent or legal guardian must sign the informed consent form. If a patient is unable to communi-

The Ohio State University
Form 9168
(465517)

The Ohio State University Hospitals

Informed request for vascular studies to be performed in the
CARDIOVASCULAR LABORATORY
Department of Radiology
410 West 10th Avenue
Columbus, Ohio 43210

Date _____ Time_____am / pm

My doctor_____, has referred me for the following

special x-ray study: _____
(nature and extent)

_____

He has informed me that the study will provide essential information, not available by other methods, concerning the nature of my illness and possible subsequent treatment.

It has been explained to me by Doctor _____.
He has also informed me and I fully understand that there are possible though infrequent serious complications which may result from these procedures, among which are _____

_____

_____

I hereby request the performance of the angiographic studies asked for by my physician, and if necessary, the use of any measures, including surgery, to alleviate possible complications that may occur. In voluntarily signing this form I acknowledge that no guaranty or assurance has been given to me by anyone as to the result which may be obtained from the performance of this study.

WITNESS: _____

(Patient's signature or person authorized to give consent for the patient)

FIG. 4-3 A typical consent form for a radiologic procedure.

cate, an interpreter must be available to explain the terms of the consent.

Because radiologic technologists are not usually the health care practitioners who perform potentially hazardous procedures, you usually will not be responsible for obtaining consent. In most institutions, this responsibility lies with the physician. However, it is your responsibility to confirm that informed consent has been obtained before beginning the procedure (Fig. 4-4).

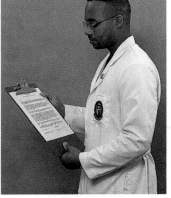

FIG. 4-4
Verify that informed consent has been given before beginning a procedure.

INCIDENT REPORTS

An **incident report** should be completed any time an event occurs that could or does result in injury to a patient or visitor. You must report all incidents of this nature, regardless of the severity of the injury. For example, an incident form should be completed if a patient falls or has a reaction to a contrast agent. Most institutions have specific forms for incidents involving patient care. Complete incident report forms quickly and do not use them to assign blame; simply document the facts.

GOOD SAMARITAN LAWS

Good Samaritan laws exist in most states to limit the legal liability of health care professionals who help someone in an emergency situation outside their usual practice setting. These laws were designed to encourage off-duty health professionals to assist in emergency situations without the fear of being sued. Good Samaritan laws offer legal immunity in emergency situations as long as health practitioners have provided the best possible care under the given conditions and have not acted beyond their scope of practice.

For example, Good Samaritan laws would protect a radiologic technologist who inadvertently breaks an automobile accident victim's rib while administering CPR. The radiographer was acting in the patient's best interest and practicing within accepted standards.

OTHER LEGAL ISSUES

The following legal issues indirectly affect the practice of radiologic technology. You should be aware of your obligations in the following circumstances.

You must report any possible cases of child abuse or sexual abuse to the appropriate authority. Pay particular attention to signs of abuse in emergency departments, because this is where you are more likely to encounter patients with abuse-related injuries. Reporting laws vary from state to state, but it is your legal obligation to know your particular state's statutes.

Legal issues also arise in the health care field when physicians make questionable treatment decisions. Physicians have the primary responsibility for directing the medical treatment of patients, and technologists are generally obligated to follow physicians' orders. However, if you believe that a physician has erred and that following an order would be detrimental to a patient's welfare, you must obtain clarification from the physician before continuing treatment. If you carry out an inaccurate order and a patient is harmed, you may be held legally responsible for that patient.

Another legal issue centers around controlled substances in the health care facility. The Comprehensive Drug Abuse Prevention and Control Act controls the distribution and administration of narcotics, depressants, stimulants, and hallucinogenic pharmaceuticals. Controlled substances may be administered only under the direction of a licensed physician and should be stored in a locked area that can only be accessed by authorized personnel. All controlled substances must also be accounted for, so any discrepancies in supplies must be reported immediately according to your institution's policies and procedures.

Although many ethical and legal challenges face health care providers, a responsible technologist who practices competently and skillfully should consider existing laws to be a positive force in radiologic technology practice. The ARRT Code of Ethics guides professional interactions with patients, family members, and other health care professionals. Understanding patients legal rights, your obligations to patients and your profession, your scope of care, and your profession's standards of practice minimizes the chance you may become involved in a lawsuit. Most important, you must dedicate your time and be personally committed to providing fair and humane treatment to all patients.

STUDY QUESTIONS

1. Explain the differences among moral values, ethics, and legal standards.
2. Choose one of the principles of professional conduct from the ARRT Code of Ethics and describe how it affects the daily working environment of a radiologic technologist.
3. Describe a situation in which a technologist may be the following:
   - Considered negligent
   - Accused of assault
   - Accused of invasion of privacy
4. Why are incident reports important in cases of patient injury?
5. Describe your state's statutes regarding reporting suspected child abuse.
6. What should you do if you suspect a physician has made an error in ordering a procedure or treatment for a patient?

Five

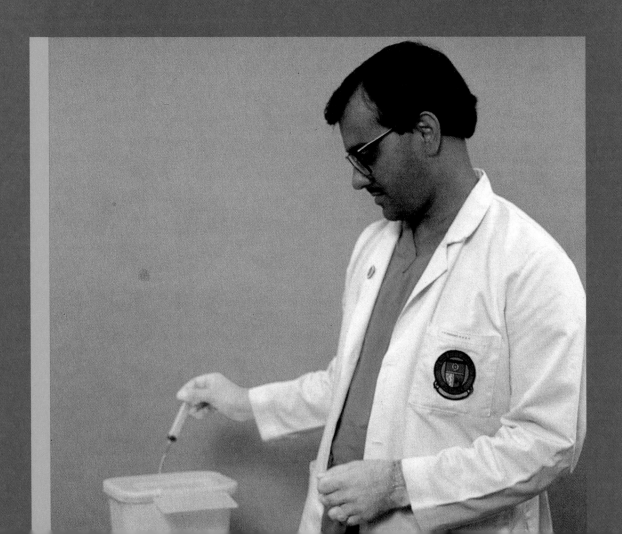

Infection Control and Aseptic Technique

Key Terms

Contents

Objectives

AFTER COMPLETING THIS CHAPTER, THE STUDENT WILL BE ABLE TO:

1. Explain how nosocomial infections can be prevented in the radiology department.
2. Diagram and explain each step in the cycle of infection.
3. Describe the Centers for Disease Control and Prevention recommendations and goals for handwashing for health care workers.
4. Explain the purpose of universal precautions and demonstrate proper universal precaution techniques.

5. List five general guidelines recommended by the Occupational Safety and Health Administration for universal precautions.
6. Define isolation precautions and explain the reason they are important to radiographers.
7. List the types of category-specific isolation and the necessary precautions for each category.
8. Demonstrate the proper procedure for radiographing a patient in isolation whether it is performed by the bedside or in the imaging department.
9. Demonstrate surgical and nonsurgical handwashing techniques.
10. Demonstrate the way to put on a sterile gown and gloves.
11. Describe at least six steps necessary for maintaining a sterile field.
12. Identify two methods of sterilizing supplies or equipment.
13. Describe the way to determine whether the contents of a package are sterile.

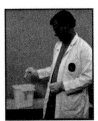 HEALTH CARE INSTITUTIONS ARE AT GREAT risk for spreading of infection and disease because of the presence of many different types of disease-causing organisms. These organisms, called *infectious microorganisms* or *pathogens*, are numerous and diverse, posing a risk to both patients and health care workers. As a health care professional, you have the responsibility to help ensure a safe, clean environment for co-workers and patients under your care. Staying healthy and recovering quickly depend in part on strict infection control. Be diligent when using infection control techniques so that you can prevent the spread of disease to patients, visitors, and co-workers.

Infectious microorganisms or pathogens entering the body cause infection. Pathogens include bacteria, viruses, fungi, and protozoa. As pathogens multiply, they affect normal tissue functions and can result in disease. Infectious microorganisms that are transmitted directly from one person to another cause contagious or communicable diseases; the common cold and AIDS are communicable diseases.

ASEPSIS

Asepsis is the state of being free from germs and results from infection control. Aseptic techniques are important for controlling the spread of infection. Radiologic technologists must practice two types of aseptic technique: medical asepsis and surgical asepsis.

Medical asepsis is also called *clean technique*. It is used to limit the number and prevent the spread of infectious microorganisms. Handwashing is the single most effective method for preventing and controlling infection. Washing hands between patients, using gloves and other protective wear, and washing hands after removing gloves help minimize the risk of transmitting microorganisms from patient to patient, patient to staff, and staff to patient. Medical aseptic technique incorporates basic principles of hygiene that should normally be practiced at home as well as in health care settings.

Surgical asepsis is also referred to as *sterile technique* because it eliminates pathogens by sterilization. Sterilization destroys microorganisms and their spores. Surgical asepsis is practiced in the operating room and where invasive procedures are performed, such as cardiovascular-interventional areas.

NOSOCOMIAL INFECTIONS

A **nosocomial infection** is an illness an individual acquires during hospitalization or while being in a hospital. As mentioned previously, hospital personnel and patients are at risk for acquiring nosocomial infections because of the hospital's large population of highly virulent microorganisms. Nosocomial infections may extend the length of patients' stays in the hospital by prolonging their recovery time, thus increasing the cost of health care. Preventing nosocomial infections is important financially and medically.

Health care workers may acquire or transmit nosocomial infections such as influenza, colds, or other infectious diseases unless strict aseptic technique is used. A patient's risk of developing a nosocomial infection depends on the number of health care workers having direct contact with the patient, the type and number of invasive procedures the patient undergoes, and the length of the patient's stay in the hospital. Patients in intensive care units are more susceptible to acquiring nosocomial infections because these units have a variety of physiologic and environmental factors that favor infection.

CYCLE OF INFECTION

For an infection to develop and be transmitted, six major components must be present (Fig. 5–1):
   1. A source (an infectious microorganism)
   2. A reservoir or medium for microorganism growth
   3. A portal of exit from the medium

4. A mode of transmission
5. A portal of entry to another individual
6. A susceptible host

For example, if a contaminated needle (portal of exit) from a patient (reservoir) with hepatitis B (source) is accidentally used (portal of entry) on another patient (susceptible host) to start intravenous therapy (mode of transmission), the chain of infection would be complete and the infection could spread from one patient to another. Because this chain is repeated, it is called the **cycle of infection**.

SOURCES AND RESERVOIRS OF INFECTION

Development of infection depends on the amount of contaminant (source) present, the type of infectious microorganism involved and its ability to grow in various conditions, and the length of time from contamination to contact with the potential host. Infectious microorganisms include bacteria, viruses, fungi, and protozoa. Common bacterial pathogens include staphylococcus, streptococcus, and *Escherichia coli*. Viral pathogens include all types of hepatitis, the herpes simplex virus, and human immunodeficiency virus (HIV).

Pathogens require nourishment and proliferate in environments such as soiled linens, contaminated water, or fluids high in glucose,

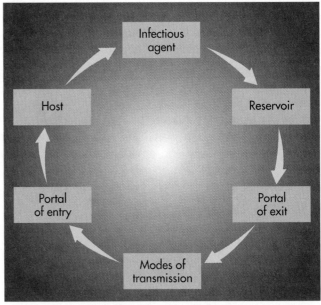

FIG. 5-1 The cycle of infection.

that encourage their growth. To grow and prosper, infectious microorganisms need food, oxygen, water, warm temperatures, an appropriate pH range, and light.

Environments conducive to pathogen survival are called *reservoirs*. Pathogens have many reservoirs suitable for growth, but the most common is the human body. Many infectious organisms live on the skin and body cavities and body fluids and discharges. Not all humans serving as reservoirs of pathogens actually become ill, however. Individuals who show no sign of illness but have infectious microorganisms in or on their bodies are called *carriers*.

Animals, insects, food, water, and inanimate objects may also be reservoirs. For instance, ticks are reservoirs for the pathogen that cause Lyme disease; mosquitos serve as reservoirs for the protozoa that cause malaria; shellfish can carry bacteria that cause cholera; and unrefrigerated milk can harbor the pathogens that cause botulism.

PORTAL OF EXIT

After infectious microorganisms grow and multiply in one site, they may pass through a portal of exit, reach another host, and spread the disease. Pathogens can leave the human body through a variety of means. The skin and mucous membranes become portals of exit when pathogens leave the body in drainage from an infected wound. The respiratory tract may be a portal of exit for microorganisms when individuals cough, sneeze, talk, or even breathe. The gastrointestinal tract is also a major source of bacterial contamination. Pathogens may be spread through saliva, feces, vomit (emesis), or bile excreted through surgical tubes and drains. Although some body systems such as the urinary tract are normally sterile, patients with urinary tract infections can spread pathogens through their urine. The blood is also normally sterile, but bloodborne pathogens such as hepatitis B use the circulatory system as their reservoir. Breaks in the skin allow pathogens to exit the body via the blood and infect susceptible hosts.

MODES OF TRANSMISSION

The next link in the chain of infection is the mode of transmission, or the way pathogens are transferred from the source to the potential new host. There are four modes of transmission: direct or indirect contact, airborne, vehicle, and vector. Many pathogens are transmitted only by certain modes, but some infectious microorganisms may be transmitted by multiple routes. If you understand the way pathogens are transmitted, you can prevent the spread of infection more effectively. Almost everything within a health care environment, including health care workers, can be a means of transporting infection.

Pathogens can be transmitted by direct or indirect contact. Direct contact is the physical transfer of the pathogen between the infected individual and the potential new host, for example, when an individual physically touches an infected patient or body fluid. Contaminated inanimate objects that have been in contact with an infected person often provide an indirect means of transmission. Infection by indirect contact occurs when an individual comes into contact with an object such as a bedpan, needle, or intravenous catheter that has been in physical contact with an infected individual. The contaminated inanimate objects capable of transmitting disease are called *fomites*.

Infection by airborne transmission occurs when an infectious pathogen in dust or droplets is inhaled. For instance, diseases such as tuberculosis, pneumonia, meningitis, and chickenpox are spread when an infected person coughs, sneezes, or breathes and disperses infectious droplets in the air. Masks worn by health care workers can prevent infection by airborne transmission.

Vehicles are inanimate items, such as water, drugs, solutions, blood, or improperly prepared or stored food, that become reservoirs for infectious microorganisms. Vehicles are different from fomites because they have not been in contact with infected individuals. A vehicle such as improperly stored food serves as a reservoir for *Salmonella* organisms. The *Salmonella* bacteria will be transmitted to the individual who eats the infected food (the vehicle).

A vector is a disease-carrying insect or animal that transmits germs to humans. A vector bites or stings an infected person and transmits the infection by biting or stinging another person. Pathogens that are commonly transmitted by vectors include malaria, Lyme disease, rabies, and typhus.

PORTAL OF ENTRY AND THE SUSCEPTIBLE HOST

Generally, pathogens do not survive very long on inanimate objects. A warm, moist environment such as the skin, however, promotes the growth of microorganisms. Pathogens can enter a susceptible host's body the same way they exit the body. For example, breaks in the skin (the body's natural protection barrier) provide portals of entry for a variety of infectious microorganisms.

All organs of the body, including the skin, have methods of defense against infection. The respiratory system, for example, has cilia, which are moving, hairlike projections that push bacteria up and out of the system. The skin has normal flora (microorganisms) that compete with infectious organisms for nourishment. Intact skin provides a substantial barrier to infection, even if it comes into contact with contaminated medical equipment.

A potential host's resistance to disease depends on several factors, including skin integrity, age (with the very young and very old having less resistance), and any underlying chronic diseases such as diabetes, immune deficiency diseases, or cancer. Certain therapeutic treatments such as radiation therapy, chemotherapy, and antibiotic therapy may also increase an individual's susceptibility to infection. In addition, particular populations are at greater risk for specific types of infection. These groups include people living in overcrowded and unclean areas, IV-drug users, and people who engage in unprotected sexual activity outside a long-term, monogamous relationship.

MEDICAL ASEPSIS

Medical asepsis techniques reduce the number of and reduce or prevent the spread of microorganisms. If the chain of infection is interrupted by medical asepsis techniques, the infection cannot spread.

Medical equipment is therefore cleaned at regular intervals with a disinfectant cleanser to prevent the transmission of pathogens among health care workers. X-ray equipment and supplies should be cleaned after use with each patient to prevent transmission of infectious microorganisms to co-workers or other patients. Bathrooms should also be cleaned after use by patients. Washing your hands between each patient contact, following universal precaution guidelines by wearing gloves and other protective wear, and washing hands after removing your gloves help prevent the transmission of infectious microorganisms.

HANDWASHING

Handwashing is the single most effective method for preventing and controlling infection. Wearing gloves does not eliminate the need for handwashing. To prevent the spread of nosocomial infections, health care workers must use good handwashing techniques (box).

Using a vigorous rubbing motion, wash your hands with an antimicrobial soap (if available) for at least 10 to 15 seconds, covering

GOALS OF HANDWASHING

- To reduce the number of transient and resident bacteria on the hands
- To prevent the transmission of infection to patients and family members
- To prevent the transmission of infection to other health care workers
- To prevent the transmission of infection to yourself

all surfaces of the wrists and hands. In settings such as surgical areas a longer handwashing routine is required.

The Centers for Disease Control (CDC) has established the following handwashing guidelines for health care workers:

Wash hands in the following situations:

1. Before contact with patients (especially if they are highly susceptible to infection)
2. After caring for infected patients
3. After touching any organic material
4. Before performing invasive procedures such as IV injections, suctioning, and bladder catheterization
5. Before and after handling dressings or touching open wounds
6. After handling contaminated equipment
7. Before preparing medications
8. Between contacts with different patients, especially those in high-risk units such as critical care and nursery units
9. After using the restroom
10. After sneezing, coughing, or blowing your nose
11. After removing your gloves

To prepare for handwashing, push your sleeves and watch above your wrists. Remove any jewelry. Stand in front of and slightly away from the sink to avoid splashing your uniform. Always assume the sink and sink handles are contaminated. Unless the sink is equipped with knee or foot controls, use a paper towel to turn water handles on and off (Fig. 5–2). If a soap dispenser is not available and bar soap must be used, always drop the soap into the soap dish or sink after lathering your hands. The soap dish should be an open-rack style to allow drainage of water and prevent buildup of soap slime, which harbors bacteria. Procedure 5-1 describes the steps of proper handwashing.

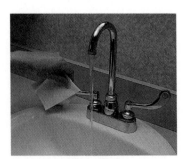

FIG. 5-2
Turn on water using a clean
paper towel.

PROCEDURE 5-1
HANDWASHING

1. Turn the water to the desired flow and temperature.
2. Wet your hands and lower your arms completely under the running water, holding hands and forearms lower than your elbows.
3. Apply a generous amount of soap to hands (1 to 2 ml).
4. Lather well (10 to 15 seconds), using friction to loosen and remove dirt and bacteria. Interlace fingers and rub palms and back of hands in a circular motion at least 5 times.

5. Use an orangewood stick to clean under and around your fingernails, being careful not to tear or cut your skin. If you wear artificial nails, spend extra time washing your hands because artificial nails may harbor more bacteria.
6. Rinse your hands and wrists thoroughly, allowing water to run from wrists to fingertips.
7. Using a paper towel, dry your hands thoroughly from fingertips to wrists and forearms. Discard the paper towel in the proper receptacle.
8. Turn the water off using foot or knee controls or a clean paper towel on hand faucet controls.

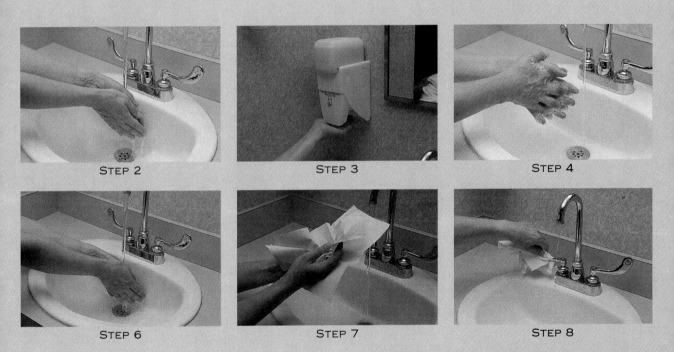

STEP 2   STEP 3   STEP 4

STEP 6   STEP 7   STEP 8

UNIVERSAL PRECAUTIONS

Because of concerns about HIV and hepatitis B infections, the CDC instituted **universal precautions** in 1987. These precautions were developed to protect health care workers from bloodborne pathogens (box).

Occupational Safety and Health Administration's (OSHA) 1991 Bloodborne Pathogens Standard defines universal precautions as the minimum standard for safety. All patients, regardless of their health history, must be considered potential carriers of bloodborne pathogens. Universal precautions should be used consistently when in contact with all patients.

Gloves are the most common type of protection used in the imaging department. Because they prevent contact with infectious organisms, gloves must always be worn when performing venipuncture, barium enema procedures, and any time your hands may come into contact with blood and body fluids. Be sure to use established handwashing techniques after removing gloves.

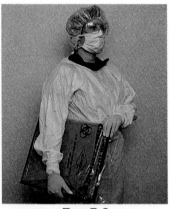

FIG. 5-3
A gown, gloves, mask, and protective eye shields must be worn when there is a likelihood of contamination with blood or body fluids.

UNIVERSAL PRECAUTIONS

- Gloves should be worn when in contact with blood, body fluids containing visible blood, mucous membranes, and nonintact skin.
- Gloves should be worn when handling items or touching surfaces soiled with blood or body fluids and when performing venipuncture and other vascular access procedures.
- Gloves should be changed after contact with each patient.
- Masks and protective eye shields should be worn during procedures that can generate droplets of blood or other body fluids to prevent exposure of mucous membranes of the mouth, nose, and eyes to infection (Fig. 5–3).
- Gowns should be worn during procedures that can result in the splashing of blood or other body fluids.
- Hands and other skin surfaces should be thoroughly washed immediately after contamination with blood or body fluids.
- Needles should not be recapped, purposely bent or broken, or removed from syringes.
- Needles and syringes must be disposed of in puncture-resistant containers in the immediate work area (Fig. 5–4).
- Mouthpieces, ambu bags, and ventilation devices should be used rather than mouth-to-mouth resuscitation.
- Health care workers with oozing or open sores should refrain from direct contact and handling patient care equipment or items.

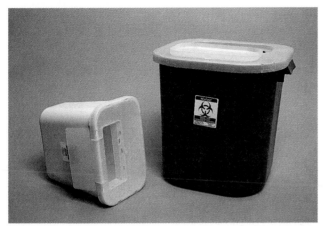

FIG. 5-4 Needles and syringes must be disposed of in puncture-proof containers.

In addition to keeping clothes from getting soiled during contact with infected patients, gowns also help prevent the spread of disease from one patient to another by health care workers. Gowns should be long enough to cover all your clothing, have long sleeves, and if possible, have tight-fitting cuffs. Discard disposable gowns after each use. Reusable gowns should be bagged according to hospital policy and laundered after each use.

Masks prevent airborne microorganisms from coming into contact with the mucous membranes of the nose and mouth. They must fit tightly over the nose and mouth and should not be reused. When a mask becomes moist, it is not an effective barrier. Change your mask periodically if it is wet. Some masks are equipped with eye guards for protection from blood and body fluid splashes.

When you are taking universal or isolation precautions and wearing a gown, gloves, and mask, remove the gloves first, then the gown, and finally the mask. Promptly wash your hands.

ISOLATION PRECAUTIONS

As a radiographer, you will encounter individuals infected with communicable diseases. **Isolation precautions** are mandated by various governmental agencies to help control the spread of pathogens that cause disease and prevent the perpetuation of the cycle of infection. Although isolation precautions are usually used to prevent the spread of disease from patient to staff or patient to patient, some patients may be placed on isolation precautions to prevent them from acquiring diseases from others. These patients have low immunities to disease because of certain health-related problems or treatments (such as patients undergoing chemotherapy) and are placed on reverse or **protective isolation** for their safety. Regulations for isolation precautions are mandated by OSHA and are strictly enforced. Recommendations regarding infection control are also issued by the CDC.

The extent of protection patients receive depends on the type of infections or diseases they have. Currently, three different types of isolation precaution control systems are in use: disease-specific isolation precautions, body substance isolation (BSI) precautions, and category-specific isolation precautions. Category-specific isolation precautions are the most commonly used isolation precautions in health care facilities. In this system the specific isolation precautions taken are determined by the category into which the patient's disease falls. These categories are described in Table 5–1.

TABLE 5-1

CATEGORY-SPECIFIC ISOLATION

CATEGORY	PURPOSE	NECESSARY ITEMS
STRICT	Prevents spread of infection through air droplets and contact	Gown, gloves, mask
CONTACT	Prevents spread of infection through direct contact	Gown, gloves, mask
RESPIRATORY	Prevents spread of infection through droplets	Mask
ENTERIC	Prevents spread of infection through direct or indirect contact with feces	Gown, gloves
TUBERCULOSIS	Prevents spread of tuberculosis	Mask, gown if necessary (for prevention of gross contamination of garments)
DRAINAGE/ SECRETION	Prevents spread of infection through direct contact	Gown, gloves

Because isolated patients are often deprived of normal social relationships, it is especially important to be friendly and caring when performing procedures. Treat patients with respect and dignity while following isolation procedures.

The nursing staff should place signs outside the doors of patients' hospital rooms and at their bedsides to remind health care workers of specific precautions to take and necessary protective gear to wear when coming into contact with patients. If you perform portable or mobile radiographic examinations on patients in isolation, you must practice medical aseptic technique.

When radiographing an isolated patient, place your lead apron under your protective gown to protect you from radiation exposure and prevent contamination of the apron. Place the cassette in a plastic bag to prevent contamination with body fluids (Fig. 5-5).

Two technologists should work together when performing what is sometimes called the *clean/contaminated technique*. The technologist that remains "clean," or uncontaminated, handles the cassette when it is outside the protective plastic bag and the portable x-ray equipment. The "contaminated" technologist has contact with the patient and cassette while it is in its protective bag (Fig. 5-6). This technologist should not touch the x-ray equipment.

Cassettes are placed in a plastic bag by the clean technologist, who passes the covered cassette to the contaminated technologist.

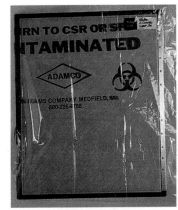

FIG. 5-5
Cassettes must be placed in a plastic bag to prevent contamination by blood or body fluids.

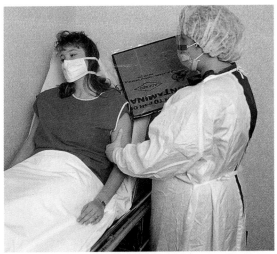

FIG. 5-6 The "contaminated" technologist handles the patient and cassette once the cassette is in the bag.

The contaminated technologist positions the cassette under the patient, and the clean technologist makes the radiographic exposure (Fig. 5-7). After the exposure has been made, the contaminated technologist takes the cassette from under the patient. The clean technologist removes the cassette from the plastic bag, being careful not to contaminate the cassette.

Anything exposed to infected material must be disinfected or discarded. Gowns, gloves, and masks should be removed and discarded in approved containers for contaminated wastes before leaving patients' rooms (Fig. 5-8). Wash your hands thoroughly after removing contaminated items, and follow any special bagging procedures used by your facility. Appropriate disposal or disinfection techniques help prevent accidental exposure of hospital personnel to infection and also prevent contamination of the surroundings.

If the mobile x-ray unit and cassette become soiled, they must be cleaned and disinfected after being removed from the patient's room. Follow the cleaning and disinfecting procedures used in your facility before returning to the radiology department or entering another patient's room.

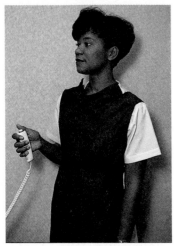

FIG. 5-7
The "clean" technologist should handle the radiographic equipment.

TRANSPORTING PATIENTS ON ISOLATION PRECAUTIONS

Patients on isolation precautions who must be transported to the radiology department should wear clean hospital gowns underneath their isolation gowns. Patients with airborne diseases should also wear regular masks. The nursing staff should notify the radiology department about patients' isolation statuses before procedures are performed so that proper technique can be followed in the imaging area. The clean/contaminated technologist procedure described previously should be followed. Items must be disinfected or discarded after contamination by the patient.

SURGICAL ASEPSIS

The goal of surgical asepsis is sterility, or the elimination of microorganisms. Sterilization is accomplished by an autoclave (steam), gas, radiation, or chemicals. Unsterile items are wrapped in sterile paper envelopes, linen, or disposable drapes. Each item is marked with an expiration date and a chemical indicator tape that becomes colored when sterilization is complete. Store sterile items in a clean, dry place. Rotate them so that similar items are used according to their expiration dates. If a package tears, opens, or becomes wet, it is contaminated.

Sterility is an absolute state—an object is either sterile or not.

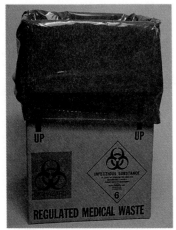

FIG. 5-8
Dispose of contaminated items properly to maintain a safe and sanitary work environment.

The slightest deviation from the described sterilization procedure causes contamination. Patients should not touch open sterile trays or drapes during procedures and should not touch body areas that have been sterilized; for example, patients should not touch their backs during myelograms. Patients should also be told not to sneeze or cough near sterile trays.

Individuals wearing sterile gloves should keep their hands above waist level. Hands lowered below the waist are considered contaminated and must be regloved to reestablish sterility.

THE STERILE FIELD

The sterile field is the area where sterile equipment is placed and the sterile procedure is performed. The technologist must be careful not to brush against, reach over, or cough or sneeze near a sterile field. The procedure room should be neat and organized. During a sterile procedure, keep the number of people in the room to a minimum. The doors should be kept closed to avoid drafts that might carry airborne pathogens. (See the box for procedures on maintaining a sterile field.)

PROCEDURES FOR MAINTAINING A STERILE FIELD

- Keep the procedure area neat and uncluttered.
- Organize all supplies before beginning the procedure to avoid interruptions.
- Avoid quick movements or rearrangement of linens after the sterile field has been opened to reduce air currents and possible airborne transmission of bacteria.
- When opening a sterile tray or adding sterile supplies to the field, minimize the number of people walking into the area.
- When opening the sterile field, wear a mask and protective hair covering. Long hair should be pulled back and fastened.
- Stand away from the sterile field when opening packages. Drop supplies onto the field without reaching over the field.
- Close doors and windows to avoid drafts.
- Only allow sterile items to touch other sterile items.
- If a sterile item touches a clean but unsterile item, it is considered contaminated.
- Do not turn away from the sterile field.
- Do not hold items below the waist or out of the field of vision because they will be considered contaminated.
- Consider the contents of any package that is torn, wet, or partially open contaminated.
- Place all sterile objects at least 2.5 cm (1 inch) from the edge of the field. The border around the outer edges of the sterile field is considered contaminated.
- Avoid touching your face or other parts of your body with sterile gloved hands.
- When pouring a sterile solution, pour out a small amount into the trash to wash bacteria from the lip of the bottle. Pour the desired amount of solution into a sterile container.

PREPARING A STERILE FIELD

You may be required to prepare a sterile field for a radiology procedure. Procedure 5-2 describes how to open a sterile, wrapped tray. Depending on the type of procedure being performed, you may be required to wear a surgical cap and mask. Many microorganisms reside in hair and can contaminate sterile objects, but if your hair is short and clean, the cap may not be necessary.

Masks prevent your respiratory system's airborne bacteria from contaminating the sterile field or a patient's exposed skin. If you have a respiratory infection, you should always wear a mask to prevent transmission of airborne bacteria (see Procedure 5-3).

Before setting up a sterile field for a procedure, wash your hands (see Procedure 5-1). After opening the tray, be sure to wear sterile gloves when handling sterile instruments and supplies (Fig. 5-9). Putting on sterile gloves (Procedure 5-4) may seem difficult initially but becomes easier the more you practice. After putting on sterile gloves, only touch sterile items. Keep your hands above waist level and avoid touching your face or clothing.

You may be required to wear a sterile gown when assisting with a sterile procedure. Before donning the sterile gown, put on the surgical cap, mask, and lead apron (if needed) and perform **surgical handwashing** (Procedure 5-5). This is also referred to as **scrubbing**. Procedure 5-6 describes how to put on a sterile gown and gloves. Technologists working in cardiovascular-interventional areas must always use surgical asepsis techniques when assisting with procedures.

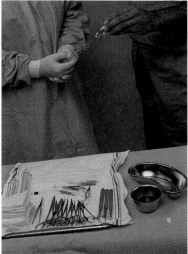

FIG. 5-9 Handle instruments with sterile gloved hands.

Text continued on p. 100.

PROCEDURE 5-2
DONNING AND REMOVING A SURGICAL MASK

A cloth or disposable paper surgical cap should be placed over the hair completely like a hair net. It should fit snugly and no hair should stick out from the edges of the cap.

Most masks are made of disposable paper. Many have metal nosepieces that bend to the contour of the nose. Put on the cap before the mask if you are going to wear both.

1. When putting on the mask, hold the top two strings or loops so that the metal nosepiece is on the top of the mask.
2. Place the nosepiece over the bridge of your nose and bend the metal slightly to fit.
3. Tie the top two strings at the back of the head (over the surgical cap if applicable) with the strings above the ears or place the loops over the ears.
4. Tie the two lower strings snugly at the nape of the neck. The front part of the mask should fit down over the chin.
5. To remove the mask, untie the lower strings first and then the top strings.
6. Remove the mask carefully, and do not drop the strings near the sterile area. Fold the mask in half with the insides together.
7. Grasp the cap at the top and lift it from your hair.
8. Discard the mask and cap in the proper receptacle and wash your hands.

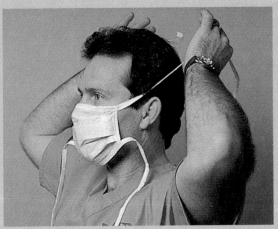

STEP 3

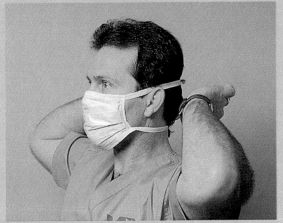

STEP 4

94

PROCEDURE 5-3
OPENING A
STERILE TRAY

1. Place the sterile tray on a sturdy, clean, flat table that is above waist level.
2. Stand away from the tray or table to avoid touching the sterile wrap with your clothes.
3. Remove the tape with the expiration date. Grasp the outer surface of the top flap of the covering. Open the flap away from you.

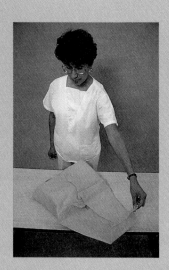

4. Grasp and open the outermost side flap. Repeat this procedure with the other side flap.

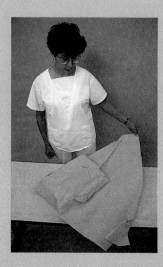

5. Open the last flap toward you, and do not touch the drape with your clothing. If the item is double wrapped, repeat this process with the inside wrap.

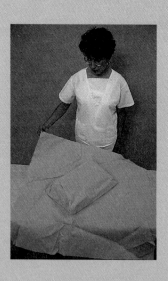

6. When the inside wrap is completely opened, the sterile field is established.

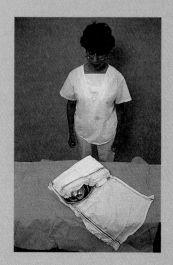

7. Sterile items may be added to the sterile field by dropping them onto the field after opening the package. Avoid reaching over the sterile field.

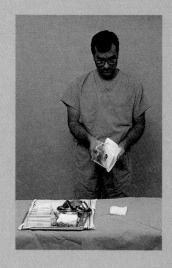

PROCEDURE 5-4
GLOVING (OPEN METHOD)

1. Put on the cap and mask if needed.
2. Perform thorough handwashing (see Procedure 5-1).
3. Open the glove wrapper carefully; start at the corner and peel back the sides.
4. Place the inner glove package on a clean, flat surface.
5. Open the package enough to identify the right and left gloves. Position the package so that the cuffs of the gloves are closest to you and the right glove is on your right side.
6. Carefully grasp the folded edges of the package and open it so that you can see the gloves.
7. Glove your dominant hand first. Grasp the glove by the cuff using the thumb and first two fingers of your nondominant hand, and lift the glove off the wrapper.

8. Pull the glove onto your dominant hand, making sure that the thumb and fingers are in the proper spaces. Leave the cuff folded.
9. Slip the first four fingers of your dominant hand under the cuff of the second glove, and slip the glove onto your nondominant hand. Be careful not to touch your ungloved hand with the dominant gloved hand or fingers. Keep the thumb of your dominant hand abducted (bent back).
10. Slip the first four fingers of your nondominant hand into the cuff of the dominant hand's glove and open the cuff over the dominant hand's wrist. Interlock your fingers to help all fingers slide completely and snugly into the gloves.
11. Wipe off any powder that is on the outside of the gloves with a wet, sterile sponge.

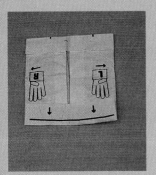

STEP 5

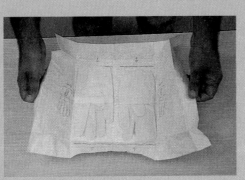

STEP 6

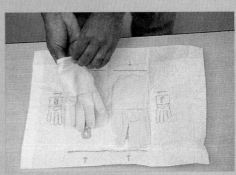

STEP 7

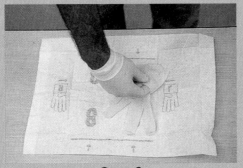

STEP 9

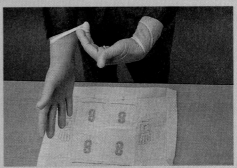

STEP 10

PROCEDURE 5-5
SURGICAL HANDWASHING

1. Cover your hair completely with the cap. Remove pierced earrings or cover them with the cap.
2. Put on the face mask, covering your mouth and nose completely.
3. Remove all jewelry, including bracelets and watches. Keep nails short and cuticles in good condition.
4. Use a deep sink equipped with knee or foot controls to dispense soap and regulate water flow and temperature. Soap should be antimicrobial; some scrub sponges are impregnated with antimicrobial soap.
5. Have two disposable hand brushes or sponges (in case one is dropped) and a disposable nail cleaner available. Impregnated sponges are often packaged with a disposable nail cleaner.

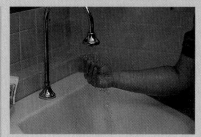

STEP 6

6. Turn the water on and adjust it to a comfortable temperature and flow; avoid splashing.
7. Wet your arms and hands well, keeping hands above elbows during the entire procedure.
8. With a liberal amount of antimicrobial soap, lather hands and arms well for a few minutes. Clean under your nails with a disposable nail cleaner.
9. Rinse your hands and arms from fingertips to elbows with running water. Keep your hands above your elbows.

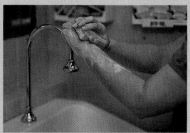

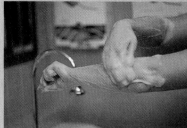

STEP 10

10. Apply soap liberally to your hands and arms to approximately 5 cm (2 inches) above the elbows with a scrub sponge or brush, using either the timed method (5 minutes per arm) or the stroke method (10 strokes to the surface of each finger, hand, wrist, and arm). Also clean your palms, the backs of your hands, and the webbed areas between your fingers.

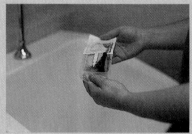

STEP 5

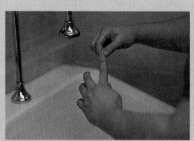

STEP 8

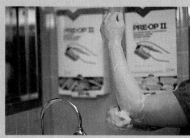

STEP 10

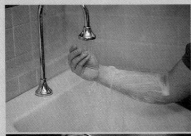

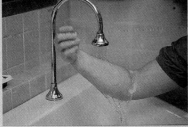

STEP 11

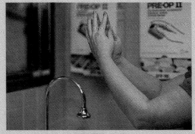

STEP 12

11. Discard the brush or sponge and rinse your hands and arms thoroughly under running water, starting at the fingertips and moving up to the elbows.

12. Allow the water to drip off your elbows.
13. Dry your hands and arms thoroughly with a dry, sterile towel, starting at the fingertips and working your way up to the elbows. Discard the towel.

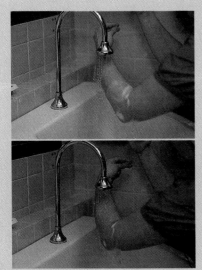

STEP 11

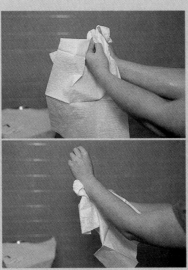

STEP 13

PROCEDURE 5-6
DONNING A STERILE GOWN AND STERILE GLOVES

1. Put on the cap, mask, and lead apron before donning the sterile gown.
2. The sterile gown will be in a paper or cloth wrap. Open the package as if opening a sterile tray (see Procedure 5-2). The gown is folded inside out so that it can be handled without contaminating the outside surface.
3. Grasp the tabs at the neck of the gown and allow the gown to unfold while holding it away from your body. The back opening of the gown should be in front of you.
4. Holding the gown at the neck opening, slide each arm into a sleeve and keep your hands inside the sleeves.

5. The neck tabs and waist tie should be secured by another, nonsterile person. The back, the area under the arms, the neckline, and the area below the waist of the gown are all considered contaminated.

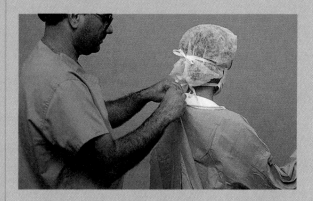

6. The package containing sterile gloves should be opened by another person and dropped onto the sterile tray.
7. With your hands inside the gown sleeves, open the side flaps of the sterile gloves.

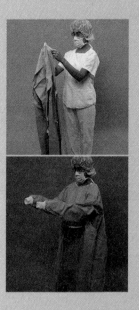

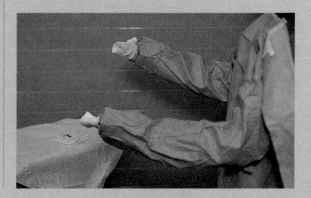

8. Using your nondominant hand inside the sleeve, lift up the glove for the dominant hand. Place the glove upside down (with the fingers of the glove pointing toward your body) on the upturned palm of the dominant hand (which is still inside the gown sleeve). The thumb of the glove should be on top of the thumb of the dominant hand (which is still inside the gown).

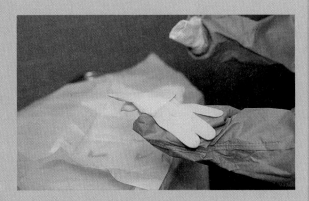

9. Using the nondominant hand, pull the cuff of the glove over the end of the dominant hand's fingers. Pulling the sleeve of the gown toward the shoulder, slide the glove onto the hand.

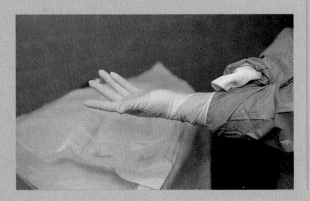

10. Pick up the other glove with the sterile gloved hand and place it upside down (as before) on the palm of the nondominant hand.

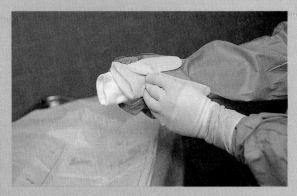

11. Pull the cuff of the glove over the fingers. Pull the gown sleeve toward the shoulder and the glove will slide onto the hand.
12. Wipe your gloved hands with a wet, sterile sponge to remove any powder. Inspect the gloves for holes or tears.

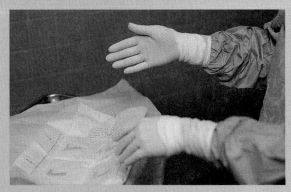

SUMMARY

In both inpatient and outpatient imaging settings, there is a risk of acquiring or transmitting infection. Knowing the links in the chain of infection allow you to intervene in and break the cycle of infection. Use universal precautions at all times, and *always* wash your hands. Prevention of infection cannot be overemphasized. Regardless of whether a particular procedure requires you to practice medical or surgical aseptic technique, all situations require you to conscientiously and knowledgeably apply infection control principles. Practice infection control daily and incorporate the procedures into your normal routines.

STUDY QUESTIONS

1. Describe the way a nosocomial infection is acquired and transmitted.
2. What are the steps in the cycle of infection?
3. How can you prevent the spread of airborne microorganisms when you have a cold?
4. Describe some of the body's mechanisms of defense against infection.
5. What factors affect a person's risk of acquiring an infection?
6. Rinsing hands with water several times each day is effective for reducing the transmission of infection. True or False?
7. When using nonsterile handwashing techniques, keep the hands below the elbows. True or False?
8. Why are isolation precautions important in your daily work?
9. List the types of category-specific isolation and the necessary protective items associated with each category.
10. What is the purpose of the clean/contaminated technologist technique?
11. Briefly explain the OSHA universal precaution regulations for health care institutions.
12. If you drop a sterile object, you can rinse it off and return it to the sterile tray. True or False?
13. Items held below the waist or out of the field of vision are considered contaminated. True or False?

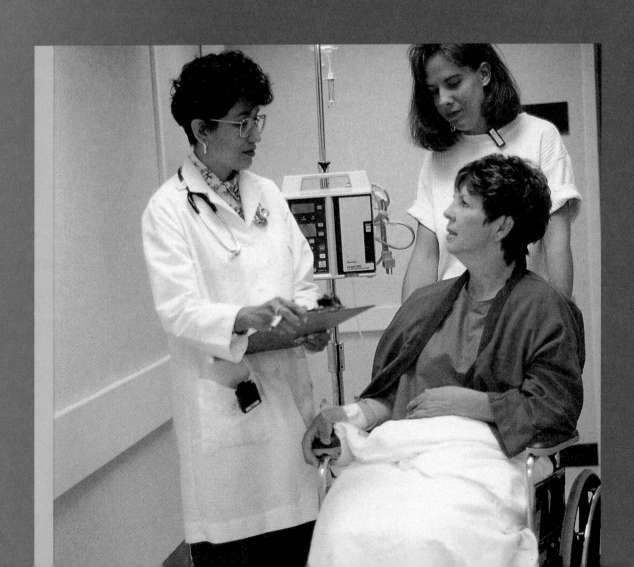

Patient Assessment and Assistance

Key Terms

Contents

Objectives

AFTER COMPLETING THIS CHAPTER, THE STUDENT WILL BE ABLE TO:

1. Describe the factors that are changing in health care and patient-focused care.
2. Identify benefits of outpatient procedures.
3. Describe Maslow's hierarchy of human needs and the way it applies to patients.

4. List the factors that influence relationships between patients and their families during a patient's illness or hospitalization.
5. Demonstrate the way to assess vital signs, including blood pressure, pulse, temperature, and respiration, and identify normal values for each.
6. Demonstrate lifting techniques using proper body mechanics.
7. Demonstrate three methods of safe patient transfer.
8. Demonstrate the way to assist patients with bedpans and urinals.

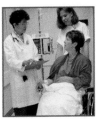

CHANGES IN THE HEALTH CARE DELIVERY system are forcing the development of a new type of patient care. Health care workers, who are being encouraged to expand their skills and job responsibilities, are able to provide patients with more individual rather than institutional care. In addition to performing imaging procedures, radiologic technologists must be able to perform a variety of patient assessment and care activities to function in their multifaceted roles.

Because today's emphasis is on patient-centered care, cross-training employees to perform core patient care activities is fairly common. Patient-centered care focuses on the patient's needs rather than the convenience of the health care provider. Radiologic technologists are often skilled in performing other imaging procedures in addition to phlebotomies and ECGs. Multiskilled professionals are able to perform a variety of patient care tasks, so fewer employees are needed to provide health care services. Professionals who have a wide range of skills are obviously more marketable than those who are trained in only one area.

Patients consider various factors when rating their overall experiences in imaging facilities. According to recent patient satisfaction surveys, these factors include the efficiency and speed of the examination, cleanliness and general appearance of the facility, and amount of explanation provided before, during, and after the examination. Patients' overall impressions are influenced by everyone with whom they come into contact.

Our first responsibility to patients is to provide them with a safe, nonthreatening atmosphere. Patients who are ill are often hypersensitive to their surroundings, so make every effort to treat them with courtesy and respect. Be comforting, empathetic, understanding, and patient.

As discussed in Chapter 2, put patients at ease by introducing yourself. Unless patients ask you to address them by their first names, address patients by "Mr." or "Ms." Look directly at patients when speaking to them. Eye contact tells patients you are sincere and have nothing to hide and will help them be more relaxed and cooperative. If you avoid eye contact, you may make patients think you are too busy to pay attention to them.

ISSUES IN AMBULATORY PATIENT CARE

Modern surgery and diagnostic testing technology has affected health care dramatically over the last decade. According to the American Hospital Association, outpatient services have steadily increased over the past 10 years. Technologic advances and increased reimbursement restrictions on inpatient care from third-party payers have led to this increase. In 1984, about 50% of all community hospitals and outpatient departments; by 1991 the number had risen to 87%.

More diagnostic and interventional radiology procedures are being done on an outpatient basis. Many free-standing outpatient facilities have opened to accommodate these changes. Many of today's patients view themselves as health care consumers, an attitude that has led to a competitive ambulatory market. Flexible scheduling, convenient locations, and attractive, comfortable decor accommodate patients' needs in settings that are less traditional than the typical hospital inpatient department. Excellent patient care and quality service are necessary to attract and maintain the patronage of modern health care consumers.

There are definite benefits to ambulatory surgery and radiology procedures. Anesthetic drugs that wear off rapidly and have fewer after-effects are used so less time is required in facilities. Ambulatory procedures also eliminate the need for hospital stays, thereby cutting costs.

Surgeons and radiologists recognize the benefits of early postoperative ambulation. They encourage patients to assume more responsibility for their own home care after they have had a procedure. Previously, inpatient care was the duty of hospital personnel. Today, when patients return home, technologists must ensure that all patients receive necessary information in both spoken and written forms. Printed instructions and department phone numbers are provided because verbal instructions can be forgotten or misunderstood in a patient's haste to be discharged.

Ambulatory and same-day procedures are challenging for technologists, nurses, and other personnel. Patients must receive detailed information about procedures in advance. The information should include risks and complications as well as pre- and postprocedure teaching instructions.

The preparation time for an ambulatory procedure is shorter than the time for an inpatient procedure, so radiology personnel must perform assessments completely and efficiently. Assessments must include patient teaching and counseling, collection and analysis of laboratory and preadmission test results, and identification of specific patient needs. The radiology nurse must also identify any risk factors for surgery or postoperative complication risk factors that the physician may have missed when taking the patient's history and performing the physical examination. The technologist should also alert the radiologist of any risk factors before the procedure (Table 6-1).

ISSUES IN INPATIENT CARE

Historically, hospitals have been the primary site for receiving health care. Patients were diagnosed, admitted, and treated and remained in the hospital until they were fully recovered. Insurance and government reimbursement policies have changed this practice. Current reimbursement policies dictate the length of time a patient may remain in the hospital for a given illness or injury (see Chapter 1 discussion of diagnostic related groups). If the patient does not recover in the predetermined length of time, alternative

TABLE 6-1

PATIENT RISK FACTORS	
RISK FACTOR	**POTENTIAL COMPLICATIONS**
Bleeding disorders (thrombocytopenia, hemophilia)	Bleeding disorders increase the risk of hemorrhaging during and after procedure.
Diabetes mellitus (DM)	DM increases the patient's susceptibility to infection and may impair wound healing. Stress caused by the procedure may cause decreased glucose tolerance.
Heart disease (recent myocardial infarction, dysrhythmia, congestive heart failure)	The stress of some procedures causes increased demands on the heart. Heart disease may increase the patient's risk for a contrast reaction.
Liver disease	Liver disease alters metabolism and the elimination of drugs that may be administered during invasive procedures.
Fever	Fever predisposes patients to fluid and electrolyte imbalances and may indicate an underlying infection.
Chronic respiratory disease	Respiratory disease may increase the patient's risk for a contrast reaction.
Immunologic disorders (leukemia, AIDS, bone marrow depression after use of chemotherapeutic drugs)	Immunologic disorders increase the risk of patient infection by health care workers and others. Wound healing is delayed after certain invasive procedures.

care must be found. Insurers often only pay for outpatient services such as diagnostic testing.

Today inpatients are usually acutely ill and may need specialized care. Many of these patients require portable or bedside procedures. Portable imaging presents multiple challenges for technologists; space limitations, radiation safety, the presence of various vascular access lines and tubes, body mechanics, and the patient's overall condition must be considered. Technologists should establish a good rapport with nursing personnel to maximize efficient, quality patient care. When performing a portable examination, for example, always speak with the nurse who is caring for the patient. You may inquire about the patient's condition, the equipment in the patient's room, or the way to position the patient without dislodging any lines. Ask for assistance with lifting the patient to avoid injury to yourself or the patient. After completing the examination, return the patient to a comfortable position. Lower the bed to its lowest position, and make sure that the siderails are up. Return any furniture that has been moved to its original place to keep aisles open and provide easy patient access.

BASIC HUMAN NEEDS

Maslow's theory of basic human needs (Fig. 6-1) helps us better understand patients. The hierarchy has five different levels. The most

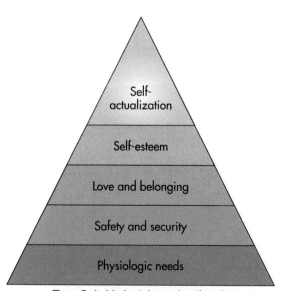

Self-
actualization

Self-esteem

Love and belonging

Safety and security

Physiologic needs

FIG. 6-1 Maslow's hierarchy of needs.

basic need is physiologic—the need for air, water, and food. The need for air can be assessed quickly by observing patients' respirations. Is their breathing unlabored? Would it help patients to sit upright or to have extra pillows? Are the patients' lips and ears pink, or are they dusky or blue? If patients are using oxygen, is it turned on and is there still an ample supply in the tank? Fulfilling the need for oxygen should have the highest priority because it is necessary for heart and brain survival.

ALERT! If a patient's respiratory history is unknown, administer 2 L O_2/min by nasal cannula (maximum) to start. Patients with chronic obstructive pulmonary disease (COPD) do not expel carbon dioxide efficiently and have altered respiration, so higher concentrations of oxygen may create more respiratory distress.

Consider the patient's hydration status. If a patient has an IV, is it dripping? Is there redness, tenderness, or swelling at the insertion site? Keep the fluid line open and intact. Patients who are in the department for routine chest x-rays or nonfasting procedures may have a sip of water if they have no other dietary restrictions.

The patient's need for food is usually not an issue in the medical imaging department. However, withholding food or requiring bowel preparation for an examination may severely deplete a patients' strength. Patients may feel weak and tired and have trouble standing or walking. When helping patients stand up, make sure their knees do not buckle and they do not get dizzy. Diabetic patients have additional problems related to fasting that are discussed later. Bowel preparation often stimulates a vasovagal response, especially in elderly patients. The signs and symptoms of a vasovagal response include hypotension (low blood pressure), pallor, vertigo (dizziness), diaphoresis (increased perspiration), and possibly syncope (fainting). Patients with heart disease are also at increased risk of having a vasovagal response because bowel preparation can also cause fluid and electrolyte imbalances.

The second basic human need is the need for physical and psychologic safety. Keeping patients physically safe includes making sure siderails are up and stretcher and wheelchair wheels are locked when transferring patients. Observe patients closely to prevent falls from tables or stretchers or while they are ambulating.

Minimizing safety risks in the medical imaging department may include transferring patients and maintaining skin integrity and body alignment. Safety risks include reactions to contrast media used in procedures, side effects of medications, and injury by equipment. Prevent equipment that comes in contact with or is used for patients from injuring patients and health care workers.

Patients' psychologic safety depends on you behaving calmly, confidently, and nonthreateningly, regardless of whether patients are confused or coherent. Many patients are unfamiliar with hospital environments, so several factors can cause anxiety.

People express anxiety in a variety of ways, including anger, withdrawal, and sarcasm. Recognize patients' anxiety and fear, and deal with them appropriately to help remove threats to psychologic safety. Providing comforting items such as blankets, pillows, sheets or pads on examining tables, and keeping bed linens flat help enhance patients' sense of security.

Maslow's third level is the need for love and a sense of belonging. Although most of us feel the need to be loved by our families and accepted by our peers, this need usually has a lower priority than physiologic and safety/security needs. People generally do not have the desire or energy to seek out or give love until they feel safe and secure.

An inpatient's family often is not present for procedures in the imaging department. However, in some outpatient settings, one or more family members may stay with the patient. To help patient's need for love and a sense of belonging, keep the family informed of the patient's status and involve them in any decision making.

Use flexible procedure scheduling to accommodate visitation times or allow time for family members to be at the hospital with patients before difficult procedures. Patients frequently want spouses or parents to be present for procedure explanations and treatments. Honor these requests as much as possible to give patients some sense of control over their situations.

Self-esteem is the fourth level in the hierarchy of human needs. Many factors may threaten a patient's self-esteem. In health care settings the change in roles is a significant factor. Sudden dependence on others, changes in body image, changes in occupational and family roles, and loss of control in decision making can all dramatically affect patients' self-esteem. To minimize this problem, maintain patients' privacy and confidentiality and treat them respectfully.

The top of Maslow's hierarchy of human needs is self-actualization or reaching your full potential. You cannot reach this level without first meeting the basic needs of the lower levels. Patients frequently cannot meet their potential because of the limitations placed on them by illness or hospitalization. As described, respecting patients' privacy, providing adequate information for decision making, and being flexible when scheduling procedures are ways in which technologists can help patients to meet their basic needs.

Basic physiologic needs take precedence over high-level needs. Different health care professionals help patients meet various needs. Understanding these needs will allow you to provide better care during routine procedures.

IMPACT OF ILLNESS ON PATIENTS AND FAMILIES

When people become ill, they progress through certain behavioral stages. If an illness is serious enough for entry into the health care system, the technologist should identify the ways in which the illness affects patients and their families.

Illness is never an isolated life event. People must deal with the changes that result not only from illnesses but from treatments as well. Each patient responds uniquely to illness, but patients and families commonly experience behavioral and emotional changes and changes in their roles, self-concepts, and family dynamics.

Environmental factors, personal behavior, and psychosocial factors all play interactive roles in illness and health. Health care professionals can no longer focus exclusively on physical health. Diagnostic assessments using complete biopsychosocial perspectives are more comprehensive. A biopsychosocial perspective encompasses all aspects of a person, including their biologic, physiologic, psychologic, and social needs.

RECORDING AND CHARTING IN THE MEDICAL RECORD

A medical record or patient chart is a written communication tool used to document comprehensive medical information about individual patients. It includes information about patients' health status and needs, as well as detailed accounts of health care services provided by physicians and other health care workers. Physicians, nurses, and other health care professionals depend on medical records to provide coordinated quality health care. Therefore, it is imperative that information entered into the record or chart is accurate and complete. Insurance companies and regulatory agencies such as the Joint Commission on Accreditation of Health Organizations (JCAHO) use medical records to determine the appropriateness and quality of care the patient has received and each health care provider's accountability in delivering the health care services. Often reimbursement from a third-party payor depends on accurate documentation of the patient's diagnosis and treatment.

Regardless of the specific recording method used, all medical records contain the following information:
1. Patient demographics
2. Consent forms

3. Medical history
4. Reports of physical examinations
5. Reports of diagnostic procedures
6. Medical diagnosis and orders
7. Progress notes
8. Nursing care plans
9. Record of patient care and treatment
10. Discharge summary

Information recorded in the medical record must be legible and written in ink. If you make an error, do not erase or block out your entry. Draw a single line through the error, write "error" above the mistake, and sign your name or write your initials. When recording patient information, begin each entry with the date and time of the entry. Record concise information and avoid unnecessary details, but also make sure all entries are complete. Enter accurate and objective information using correct spelling and proper medical abbreviations. Never include critical comments about patients or other health care professionals. Information must be factual and should be organized in a logical format. Record only for yourself and never for someone else, and do not leave blank spaces in your notes. Draw a line horizontally through any empty space and end the entry with your signature and title.

Optimum recording requires that each entry is the following:
1. Accurate: The information must be correct and precise
2. Concise: Keep the information brief and avoid unnecessary words and details; use proper abbreviations
3. Thorough: All entries must be complete
4. Current: Write the date and time of each entry
5. Organized: Record information in a logical order
6. Confidential: The law protects patient information

ASSESSING VITAL SIGNS

Radiologic technologists must be able to perform basic procedures such as measuring blood pressure, pulse, temperature, and respirations. They should also know the normal values for each of these **vital signs** (box). A patient's vital signs can deviate from the normal ranges listed, so refer to the individual's baseline vital signs in the chart to note any changes.

In patient's charts the most recent vital signs are usually recorded on graph paper. Vital signs may reveal sudden changes in patients' conditions that should be reported to a physician. Changes like these may indicate the need for additional medical care. The box describes when to take vital signs.

NORMAL ADULT VALUES FOR VITAL SIGNS

TEMPERATURE

Oral: 98.6° F (±1° F), 37° C
Rectal: 99.6° F, 37.6° C
Axillary: 97.6° F, 36.4° C

PULSE

Infant: 100 to 180 beats/min
Child: 70 to 110 beats/min
Adult: 55 to 90 beats/min

RESPIRATORY RATE

12 to 20 breaths/min

BLOOD PRESSURE

Average: 120/80 mm Hg (systolic/diastolic)
Hypertension:
 Systolic blood pressure above 140 mm Hg
 Diastolic blood pressure above 90 mm Hg
Hypotension: Systolic blood pressure below 90 mm Hg with signs of
 dizziness and increased pulse rate
Orthostatic hypotension: Decrease of 25 mm Hg in systolic blood
 pressure and 10 mm Hg in diastolic blood pressure accompanied
 by symptoms of inadequate cerebral perfusion when moving from
 lying position to sitting or standing position.

WHEN TO TAKE VITAL SIGNS

TAKE VITAL SIGNS IN THE FOLLOWING SITUATIONS:

When the patient is admitted to the health care facility
Before and after any interventional or invasive diagnostic procedure
Before and after administering any medications (including contrast
 media) that may affect cardiovascular, neurologic, respiratory, and
 temperature function
Any time the patient's general condition changes, for example, they
 lose consciousness, bleed, or have increased pain
Whenever the patient reports symptoms of distress, such as dizziness, shortness of breath, or "feeling funny."

Blood pressure is the force exerted by the blood against the vessel wall. The standard units for measuring blood pressure are millimeters of mercury (mm Hg). This measurement represents the height to which the blood pressure can raise a column of mercury in a sphygmomanometer. During a normal cardiac cycle, the blood pressure reaches a peak, or high point, and then a low point. The peak is the maximum pressure exerted against the arterial wall and occurs during **systole** (the contraction phase) as the left ventricle pumps blood into the aorta. The trough (low point) of minimum pressure occurs during **diastole** (the rest phase) as the ventricles relax. Diastolic pressure is the minimum pressure exerted against the arterial walls at all times. The blood pressure is recorded with the systolic reading over the diastolic reading (for example, 110/70).

BLOOD PRESSURE EQUIPMENT

A **sphygmomanometer** is a device for determining liquid pressure. This pressure manometer has an occlusive cloth cuff enclosing an inflatable rubber bladder, which is inflated by a pressure bulb with a release valve. There are two types of manometers: aneroid and mercury (Fig. 6-2).

The aneroid manometer is a glass-enclosed gauge containing a needle that registers millimeter calibrations. Before using an aneroid manometer, be sure the needle points to zero and the instrument is correctly calibrated. The mercury manometer is an upright tube containing mercury. Pressure created by inflation of the cuff moves the column of mercury upward against the force of gravity. Millimeter calibrations mark the height of the mercury column.

Cuffs come in several sizes ranging from small pediatric cuffs to extra-large cuffs that are used for obtaining femoral blood pressure.[5] The correct size cuff should always be used to ensure an accurate reading. The cuff should be approximately 20% wider than the circumference of the limb on which the cuff is being placed. If the cuff is too small it will not stay in place during inflation; if it is too large, it will not adequately prevent blood flow to the extremity and will result in an inaccurate blood pressure reading.

A stethoscope (Fig. 6-3) is used to **auscultate** or detect sound waves created by the arterial pulse. The four major parts of the stethoscope are the earpieces, binaurals, tubing, and chestpiece.

The chestpiece is composed of a bell and diaphragm. The diaphragm is the circular, flat portion of the chestpiece that has a thin plastic disk. The diaphragm is generally used for listening to the blood pressure. The bell is the cone-shaped portion of the chestpiece. It transmits low-pitched sounds such as heart and vascular

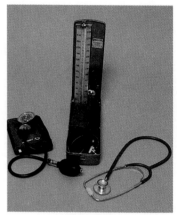

FIG. 6-2
Aneroid *(left)* and mercury *(right)* manometers.

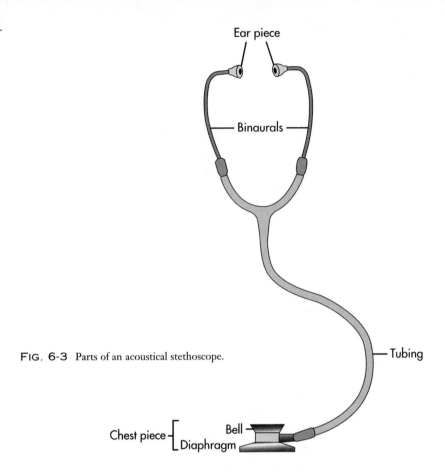

Fɪɢ. 6-3 Parts of an acoustical stethoscope.

sounds. You can use either the bell or the diaphragm by rotating them into position on the chestpiece as needed.

Determine the best site for blood pressure assessment by palpating (feeling with your fingers) for an arterial pulse. Do not apply a blood pressure cuff to an arm under the following circumstances: when an IV is in the antecubital fossa and IV fluids are infusing, in the presence of an arteriovenous shunt, when breast surgery has been performed on the side of the arm you will use, or if there is severe edema. Procedure 6-1 describes the steps for assessing blood pressure.

BLOOD PRESSURE ABNORMALITIES
In patients with certain diseases such as arteriosclerosis, the arterial walls lose their elasticity as normal tissue is replaced by fibrous tissue that does not stretch as easily. Reduced elasticity creates more resistance to blood flow. As blood is forced through rigid arterial

1. Wash your hands.
2. Explain the procedure to the patient.
3. Have the patient sit or lie down with the forearm supported at the level of the heart and the palm of hand turned up (see illustration).
4. Expose the upper arm by removing any constricting clothing.
5. Palpate the brachial artery.
6. Position the cuff 2.5 cm (1 inch) above the site of the brachial artery (antecubital space). Center the bladder of the cuff above the artery.

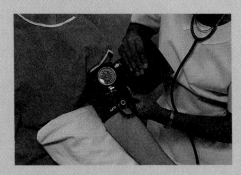

7. Wrap the fully deflated cuff evenly and snugly around the upper arm.

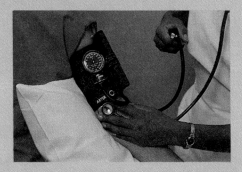

8. Be sure the manometer is positioned so that it is easily visible.
9. Palpate the brachial or radial artery with the fingertips of one hand while using the other hand to inflate the cuff rapidly to 30 mm Hg above the point at which the pulse disappears.

Slowly deflate the cuff and note the point at which the pulse reappears.

10. Deflate the cuff fully, and wait 30 seconds to prevent venous congestion and false high readings.
11. Place the stethoscope earpieces in your ears, and be sure the sounds are clear, not muffled. If you cannot hear any sounds, make sure you are using the diaphragm and not the bell of the stethoscope.
12. Relocate the brachial artery and place the diaphragm over it.
13. Close the valve of the pressure bulb by turning it clockwise until it is tight.

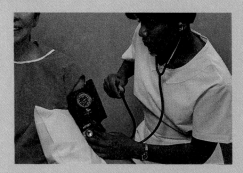

14. Inflate the cuff to 30 mm Hg above the patient's normal systolic level.
15. Slowly release the valve, allowing mercury to fall at a rate of 2 to 3 mm Hg/s.
16. Note the point on the manometer at which the first clear sound is heard. This is the systolic blood pressure.
17. Continue to deflate the cuff gradually, noting the point at which the sound becomes muffled or disappears. This is the diastolic blood pressure.
18. Deflate the cuff rapidly and remove it from the patient's arm unless you need to repeat the procedure. If this is necessary, wait 30 seconds before proceeding (venous congestion may produce a false-high reading).
19. Inform the patient of the reading.
20. Assist the patient with returning to a comfortable position and re-cover the upper arm if it was previously clothed.
21. Wash your hands.
22. Record the findings in the patient's chart or radiology department records according to your departmental standards.

walls, the blood pressure rises. This increase in blood pressure is called **hypertension.** Hypertension is a major cause of death, heart attacks, and strokes in the U.S. and Canada. Hypertension in adults is diagnosed in two different ways. With either method the patient's blood pressure is taken during at least two separate visits to the doctor.

One method measures the diastolic (minimum) pressure. When an average of two or more diastolic readings is 90 mm Hg or higher, the patient is diagnosed with hypertension. The second method measures the systolic (maximum) pressure. When an average of two or more systolic readings is consistently higher than 140 mm Hg, the patient is diagnosed with hypertension.

Remember that both methods require multiple visits to the doctor and multiple blood pressure readings during each visit. One elevated blood pressure recording does not mean a patient has hypertension. While a patient is in the imaging department, several factors may cause a temporarily elevated blood pressure, such as fear, anxiety, pain, and fluid overload.

If patients have an abnormally low pressure when they sit or stand, they have **orthostatic hypotension**. This type of low blood pressure may result from the effects of drugs or **hypovolemia** (a diminished blood supply). An acute hemorrhage following a trauma is a common cause of hypovolemic shock, but this form of shock may also be caused by a large loss of body fluids. Fluids may be lost following thermal injuries such as burns or from the gastrointestinal tract after excessive vomiting or diarrhea. Fluid may also pool within the peritoneal cavity after a gastrointestinal tract perforation and result in hypovolemia. Hypovolemic shock may also result from hypersensitivity to substances such as contrast agents that are used in radiology. Common symptoms include feeling faint or lightheaded, having visual blurring, and sudden syncope. Any change in blood pressure should immediately be reported to a physician. The appropriate medical intervention depends on the cause of abnormality.

TEMPERATURE

The hypothalamus normally regulates the body's temperature to within 0.6° C above or below 37° C (98.6° F). Temperatures outside the normal range may result from disease, infection, exercise, prolonged exposure to heat or cold, or hormonal disturbances. The body attempts to adjust to temperature changes by conserving or losing heat as needed. **Pyrexia** is the medical term for fever.

Temperature assessments are rarely used in imaging departments. However, you may be asked to perform this task. The easiest way to obtain an accurate temperature reading is orally using a thermometer. Do not use this method, however, if patients may injure themselves by biting down on the glass thermometer or if they are unable to hold the thermometer under their tongue with their lips closed long enough to ensure an accurate reading. Wait 20 to 30 minutes after patients have eaten hot or cold foods or smoked before taking their temperature. These factors can cause false temperature readings.

TYPES OF THERMOMETERS

The three types of thermometers most commonly used are mercury-in-glass, electronic (Fig. 6-4), and disposable. The common, inexpensive mercury-in-glass thermometer consists of a sealed glass tube with a mercury-filled bulb at one end. Warming the bulb causes the mercury to rise in the tube. The length of the thermometer is marked with Fahrenheit or centigrade calibrations (Fig. 6-5). These types of thermometers must be disinfected with a chemical solution after each use and are no longer commonly used in most medical facilities.

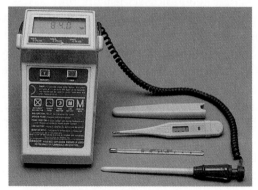

FIG. 6-4 Glass and electronic thermometers.

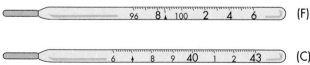

(F)

(C)

FIG. 6-5 Mercury-in-glass thermometers calibrated in centigrade and Fahrenheit.

The electronic thermometer works quickly and is easy to use. It consists of a battery-powered display unit, a thin wire cord, a temperature-sensitive probe, and disposable plastic sheaths that cover the probe and are discarded following each use. Each unit usually comes with two probes—a blue probe for oral and axillary use and a red probe for rectal use. Body temperature can be measured in seconds. Because the electronic thermometer is not made of glass, breakage is not a danger, and the disposable plastic sheaths minimize the risk of infection.

Disposable, single-use thermometers are thin strips of plastic with chemically impregnated paper used for oral or axillary temperatures. Chemical dots on the thermometer change colors to reflect temperature readings, usually within 45 seconds. The highest-numbered dot indicates the patient's temperature. These thermometers are used only once and discarded, decreasing the chance of spreading infection.

The tympanic-membrane thermometer is relatively new. It consists of a temperature-sensitive probe that is placed in the opening of the ear canal. The blood flow near the tympanic membrane warms the probe, and within seconds the unit registers the patient's temperature. Although this thermometer may be used with patients of any age, it is especially helpful for assessing the temperature of pediatric patients.

Since radiologic technologists usually only assess oral and axillary temperatures, rectal temperature will not be discussed. If there are reasons patients cannot have their oral temperatures taken, such as they can only breathe through their mouth, or they are on oxygen, the axillary method is usually used. An axillary temperature is less accurate than oral and rectal temperatures, however, because the thermometer is placed on the skin and measures the external body temperature instead of the internal body temperature.

An axillary temperature reading is typically lower than the patient's actual temperature. Procedures 6-2 and 6-3 describe the steps for taking oral and axillary temperatures with glass thermometers.

PULSE

A **pulse** is produced each time the left ventricle of the heart contracts and forces blood into the aorta and peripheral arteries. This pulse wave can be palpated by lightly pressing the artery against underlying bones or muscles. The most common site to palpate the pulse is the radial artery. Other easily accessible sites include the brachial, carotid, and axillary arteries. In life-threatening situations

PROCEDURE 6-2
TAKING AN ORAL TEMPERATURE WITH A MERCURY-IN-GLASS THERMOMETER

1. Wash your hands.
2. Help the patient obtain a comfortable position.
3. Make sure the thermometer is clean and that the mercury reads below 35.5° C (96° F). If the mercury is above the desired level, grasp the upper end of the thermometer securely, and stand away from any solid objects. Sharply flick your wrist downward as if you are cracking a whip. Continue until the mercury is at the desired level.
4. Insert the thermometer into the patient's mouth under the tongue. Ask the patient to hold the thermometer with lips closed.
5. Leave the thermometer in place 2 to 3 minutes or for the amount of time designated by your institution's policy.
6. Carefully remove the thermometer, and read it at eye level.
7. Wipe the thermometer with a tissue, and dispose of the tissue. Wash the thermometer in warm soapy water, rinse it with cool water, and let it dry. Store the thermometer in its container after shaking the mercury down again.
8. Record the temperature and method of measurement in patient's chart.

PROCEDURE 6-3
TAKING AN AXILLARY TEMPERATURE WITH A MERCURY-IN-GLASS THERMOMETER

1. Wash your hands.
2. Help the patient obtain a comfortable position, and close the curtains to ensure privacy.
3. Remove the gown or clothing from the patient's shoulder or arm.
4. Make sure that the mercury is at the desired level. (If it is at a level that is higher than normal, shake it down as described in Procedure 6-2.)
5. Place the bulb end of the thermometer in the center of the patient's axilla. Lower the patient's arm over the thermometer, and place the patient's forearm across the chest.
6. Hold the thermometer in place for 5 to 10 minutes or for the amount of time designated by your institution's policy.
7. Carefully remove the thermometer and read it at eye level.
8. Assist the patient with replacing the gown or clothing.
9. Wipe off the thermometer with a tissue and dispose of the tissue. Wash the thermometer in warm soapy water, rinse it with cool water, and let it dry. Store the thermometer in its container after shaking the mercury down again.
10. Record the temperature and the method of measurement in the patient's chart.

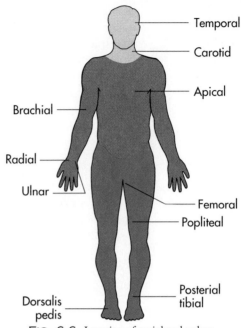

FIG. 6-6 Location of peripheral pulses.

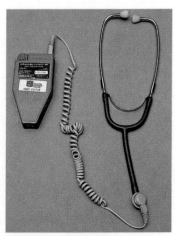

FIG. 6-7
Doppler device for obtaining pulse.

a patient's peripheral blood flow may be greatly reduced to maintain blood supply to the brain, thereby diminishing the peripheral pulses. If peripheral pulses are not detectable, take the carotid artery pulse. The carotid pulse is usually the last pulse to diminish and cease during a cardiac arrest.

The patient's pulse provides valuable information about the cardiovascular system. An abnormally slow, rapid, or irregular pulse may indicate any one of several medical problems. The strength of the peripheral pulses also may indicate whether an adequate blood supply is reaching the extremities (See Fig. 6-6 for locations of the peripheral pulses). Procedure 6-4 describes the steps for assessing a radial pulse.

If the pulse is not easily palpated, a **Doppler** ultrasound device (Fig. 6-7) may be used to auscultate the pulse. This special stethoscope contains a transducer that transmits the amplified sound waves produced by the blood flowing through the artery. A special gel is used on the skin to provide better contact with the transducer for picking up the sound waves. A whooshing sound indicates arterial blood flow. Doppler devices are commonly used in intensive care units and cardiovascular interventional laboratories.

PROCEDURE 6-4
MEASURING RADIAL PULSE

1. Wash your hands.
2. If available, determine the previous baseline rate from the patient's chart.
3. If the patient is supine, place the patient's forearm across the lower chest with the wrist extended and the palm facing down. This ensures a relaxed arm position and full artery exposure for palpation. If the patient is seated, support the lower arm on the chair or your arm.
4. Place the tips of your first two or middle three fingers over the groove along the radial side (thumb side) of the patient's inner wrist.

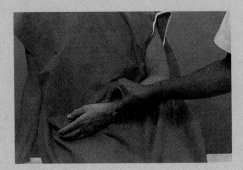

5. Lightly press your fingers against the radius. When you feel a regular pulse, look at your watch's second hand and begin to count the pulse rate: when the second hand reaches a number on a dial, count starting with zero, then continuing with one, two, three, and so on.
6. If the pulse is regular, count the rate for 15 s and multiply it by four to obtain the total beats/min.
7. If the pulse is irregular, count the rate for 1 full min.
8. Record the rate, regularity, and strength of the pulse. For example: HR-76, regular, strong; or HR-100, irregular, weak. (HR is the abbreviation for the heart rate, which is measured by the pulse.)

RESPIRATIONS

Carbon dioxide and oxygen are exchanged between the alveoli and red blood cells in the lungs. This process is called **respiration**. The lungs are also responsible for the perfusion (distribution) of blood through the pulmonary capillaries.

When you assess a patient's respirations, you observe and record the breathing rate, depth, and rhythm. Little effort is needed to inhale, and less is needed to exhale. When patients have breathing difficulties, however, they use their intercostal and accessory muscles and produce more pronounced movements of the shoulder,

1. Be sure the patient is in a comfortable position, because discomfort can cause the patient to breathe more rapidly.
2. Place the patient's arm across the abdomen or lower chest, or place your hand directly on the patient's upper abdomen. You may use the same position used for pulse measurements, especially if measuring pulse at the same time. This makes respiration measurements less conspicuous.
3. Observe a complete respiratory cycle (one inspiration and one expiration).
4. After observing a cycle, begin to count the rate when your watch's second hand hits a number on the dial; count "one" to begin the first full cycle.
5. For adults, count the number of respirations taken in 30 s and multiply by two; count the respirations for 1 min if they are irregular, very slow, or very fast. For infants or young children, count for 1 full minute.
6. While counting, note the depth, symmetry, and ease of respirations.
7. Record results in the patient's chart. For example: Resp. -20, normal depth, even and unlabored; or Resp. -32, shallow, even and labored.

neck, and chest muscles. Procedure 6-5 describes the steps for measuring respirations.

Sudden changes in a patient's respiration rate, depth, or rhythm indicate respiratory distress and should be reported immediately to a physician. If left untreated, respiratory failure may result. Respiratory depression or a lack of oxygen affect the cellular metabolism of the body organs (referred to as *cellular hypoxia*), which in turn depresses breathing and circulation and can lead to respiratory arrest. If oxygen deprivation to body organs is severe, irreversible damage may occur in minutes. A lack of oxygen to the tissues results in cyanosis, a bluish-gray discoloration of the skin. Cyanotic patients require immediate medical attention.

MOVING AND POSITIONING PATIENTS

BODY MECHANICS

Health care workers frequently suffer back injuries because of improper lifting or moving techniques. Your responsibility to your employer, yourself, and the patient is to use the principles of proper body mechanics to prevent injuries and ensure the safety of the patient and yourself.

Good body mechanics comprise balancing, aligning, and moving properly. The first principle, proper balance, involves your base of support. Having a broad base of support means that you space your

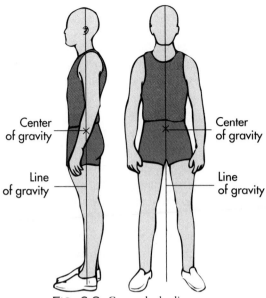

FIG. 6-8 Correct body alignment.

feet so your body is balanced when you are standing. When your body is off balance, it will lean or fall because of gravity. Your center of gravity, the point around which your body weight is balanced, is an important aspect of proper balance. Body weight is usually centered in the lower abdomen or pelvis, but when you lift an object, its weight alters your center of gravity. You need to keep your center of gravity close to the center of your base of support to maintain good balance (Fig. 6-8).

The second body mechanics principle is body alignment, or posture. When lifting, keep your back straight, bend your knees, and avoid twisting because it severely strains the spine. Keep the object close to your body (your center of gravity) and balanced over both feet, which should be parallel and slightly apart. Work at a comfortable height whenever possible, and keep your head erect.

The third and final principle concerns movement. Use the abdominal and leg muscles rather than the muscles of your lower back to lift heavy objects. If you bend over to lift an object rather than bending your knees and squatting, you risk straining your back muscles and injuring your lumbar spine. Roll or push heavy objects whenever possible, and lift them only when absolutely necessary. When lifting heavy objects or moving patients from stretchers to tables, use smooth, steady movements to help prevent back injuries.

ASSISTING WITH DRESSING AND UNDRESSING PATIENTS

Most outpatients undergoing imaging procedures do not require direct assistance putting on and taking off gowns. However, it is important to explain the way the gown should be orientated before leaving patients to dress themselves. Specify whether the gown should tie in the front or the back. Explain where all the ties and velcro tabs fasten. Explain the reason there are three sleeves in certain gowns. Hospital gowns come in a variety of styles, so be sure to assist patients with fastening gowns to ensure adequate coverage and maintain their dignity. In addition, offer patients a robe and slippers, especially if they must walk in public hallways to reach the imaging room.

Pediatric, geriatric, acutely ill, and emergency department patients may require direct assistance with putting on and taking off gowns for procedures. A family member may assist them with dressing and undressing. Be sure to instruct family members on correct gown placement. If a patient has reduced mobility or an injury to an extremity, begin by removing clothing from the unaffected side of the body. When dressing the patient, always begin clothing the affected side first. Maintain the patient's privacy and dignity at all times.

If a patient has an IV in place, remove clothing from the side without the IV first, lower the IV bag, and slide the sleeve over the patient's arm and IV. When dressing a patient with an IV, reverse this process by first placing the IV through the sleeve of the gown. Slide the arm with the IV through the sleeve followed by the arm without the IV.

TRANSFERRING PATIENTS

Patients who have not been out of bed for a length of time or are unable to stand safely should be transported by stretcher. Stretcher transport can prevent fatigue and possible injury to patients, especially those who will spend a long time in the imaging department. If patients must stand or sit for an examination, help them into a sitting position slowly; let them rest before proceeding further. Remember that patients who have been restricted to bed rest will often experience orthostatic hypotension when placed in an erect position.

Assess patients' physical health to determine whether any neurologic conditions such as numbness, weakness, or paralysis exist. You must determine patients' ability to bear weight on their legs before helping them stand for any examination or transferring them to examination tables.

When transferring and positioning patients, be careful not to bump or tear their skin. Patients with circulatory or nutritional problems are especially susceptible to skin breakdown. Patients receiving anticoagulant (blood thinning) medications are more prone to bruising and bleeding.

Patients with urinary or fecal incontinence must be kept clean and dry to prevent skin irritation, which could lead to ulcer formation.

TRANSFER FROM STRETCHER TO TABLE

If patients can move without assistance, be sure they understand the transfer procedure. All objects such as overhead x-ray tubes must be out of the patient's way. Lock the wheels of the stretcher, lower the siderails, and position at least one staff person against the stretcher to prevent its movement away from the table. Try to position another person on the other side of the table to help the patient move onto it.

If patients cannot move without assistance, transfer them with sheets or slide boards. Begin by telling patients the steps you will take during the transfer. This will prevent a fear of falling when patients are moved. If a sheet is used, have at least four people assisting you—two against the cart and two on the other side of the table. Position one person at the patient's head and one at the patient's feet to guide and support the patient and help keep the patient's body in proper alignment.

Loosen the sheet from the mattress and roll it close to the patient's body so that it can be grasped easily (Fig. 6-9). Be sure that IV lines, oxygen tubing, and urinary catheters are free and will not be pulled during the transfer. Make sure that the head and feet move in alignment with the body and are not bumped. Ask patients to hold their heads up during the transfer (to avoid bumping) if they are awake and able to do so. Coordinate the transfer by counting to three and moving in unison. Always keep the patient covered.

TRANSFER USING A SLIDE BOARD

If available, always use a slide board to transfer patients who cannot move without assistance from a cart to a table or vice versa. The slide board creates a smoother, more uniform transfer with little or no discomfort. Slide boards also provide easier transfers for trauma and obese patients, and they reduce the number of people needed to perform the transfer. At least one person should be on each side of the patient. To use a slide board, use the sheet underneath the pa-

A

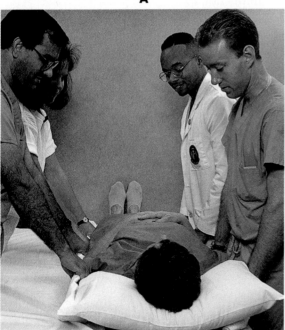

B

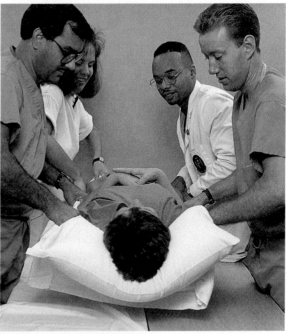

C

FIG. 6-9 Patient transfer using a sheet.

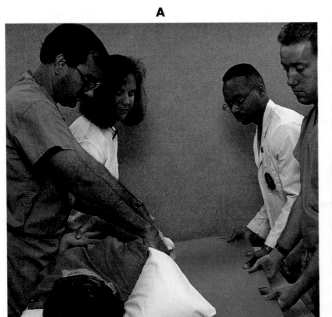
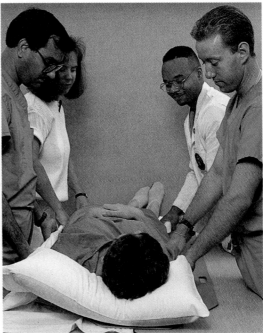

FIG. 6-10 Patient transfer using a slide board. **A,** Log roll the patient to one side and position the slide board. **B,** Slide the patient onto the slide board.

tient to roll the patient, as if you were rolling a log, away from the table (Fig. 6-10, *A*). Keep the patient's body aligned. Slide the board underneath the sheet as far as possible. Return the patient to the supine position with the sheet and board underneath. Roll the sheet up close to the body and instruct the patient to cross the arms over the chest. Count to three in unison and slide the patient onto the table (Fig. 6-10, *B*).

Radiolucent slide boards may be left under the patient during short examinations. If the board must be removed, reverse the procedure by using the sheet to roll the patient the opposite way and remove the board. After returning patients to stretchers, make sure that linens lie flat underneath them, lines and tubes are not tangled and are intact, and the patient is covered. Always raise the siderails and secure any straps.

TRANSFER TO AND FROM A WHEELCHAIR

Explain the transfer procedure to the patient before you begin transferring. IV poles and overhead x-ray tubes should be out of the way, and the floor should be dry. The patient should wear slippers. If moving the patient out of a wheelchair, place the chair parallel to

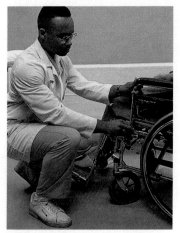

FIG. 6-11
Lock the wheelchair's wheels.

the table. Lock the wheels (Fig. 6-11), lift the footrests out of the patient's way, and place a step stool next to the table.

Even though patients may be competent and able to move independently, offer them assistance by standing beside them and placing one hand beneath their elbow. A patient may appear healthy but still be weak from an illness, surgery, or prolonged bed rest. For patients' safety, always offer them assistance when they leave the chair. (*Note*: If the patient has a weak side, assist on this side to ensure stability.)

If the patient has an IV, is on oxygen, or has a urinary drainage or reservoir bag, make sure that all tubing moves with the patient and that urinary drainage bags stay lower than the patient's bladder. The patient should step onto the stool (Fig. 6-12, A) and pivot to put the back toward the table. The patient should then sit down on the table (Fig. 6-12, B). Help the patient lie down, and place an arm underneath the shoulders while lowering the patient to the table. A second person may be needed to lift the legs and swing them up onto the table as you lower the upper half of the patient's body while at the patient's head.

If the patient cannot get into a standing position from the wheelchair, see Procedure 6-6 for assisted transfer methods.

Once the examination is complete, reverse the transfer procedure to return the patient to the wheelchair. Be sure to lock the wheels and lift the footrests before moving the patient. Provide support for patients as they ease back into the chair.

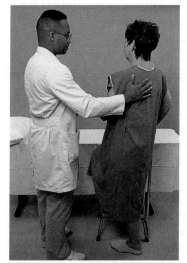
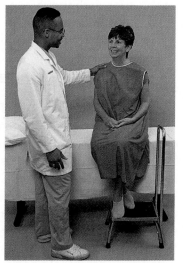

FIG. 6-12 **A,** Help patient step on stool. **B,** Patient turns around with back to table and sits down on table.

PROCEDURE 6-6
ASSISTED TRANSFER
FROM A WHEELCHAIR

1. Place the chair parallel to the table, lock the wheels, and lift the footrests out of the way. Make sure that the step stool is next to the table.
2. Stand between the footrests, facing the patient. Keep your back straight, bend your knees, and place your arms underneath the patient's arms with your hands on the patient's back.
3. Have the patient lean slightly forward. Using a rocking motion, on the count of three help the patient into a standing position. Straighten your back as the patient stands. Your legs should do most of the work. Do not proceed unless the patient is balanced.
4. Assist the patient to a stool or table, depending on the type of procedure being performed.

POSITIONING PATIENTS

The technologist should cover the table with a sheet to prevent skin burns or tears as the patient slides onto the table. For a longer examination, use a radiolucent pad. Place sponges or pads beneath the patient's knees or anywhere else support is needed (Fig. 6-13).

For thin or elderly patients, pad bony prominences for patient comfort and to avoid ulceration resulting from pressure. Periodically help the patient change positions during extended studies to relieve pressure.

Placing pillows under patients' heads provides additional comfort and may assist patients who have difficulty breathing while lying down. If patients become short of breath or cyanotic when lying down, help them sit up immediately. If patients are feeling nauseous, roll them to their sides, or help them sit up to prevent aspiration of emesis if they vomit.

X-ray tables are not equipped with siderails, so use safety straps or compression bands to prevent falls from the table. Patients with an altered state of consciousness because of sedation, senility, neurologic dysfunction (such as seizure disorders), or intoxication should not be left alone on the x-ray table even when straps or compression bands are in place. Before and after procedures, all patients lying on carts should have both or all siderails up (Fig. 6-14).

HELPING PATIENTS WITH ELIMINATION NEEDS

While in the imaging department, patients may need to urinate or defecate. Patients may be uncomfortable or embarrassed about re-

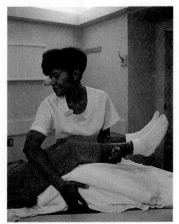

FIG. 6-13
Provide support under the patient's knees to relieve back strain.

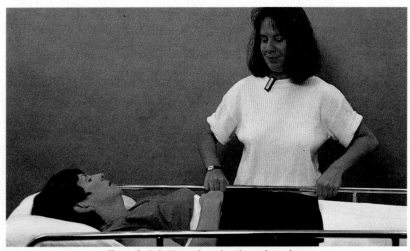

FIG. 6-14 Keep the siderails up for safety.

questing assistance, and they may avoid asking for help until their need is urgent. Accommodate a patient's request as quickly as possible to prevent further discomfort or possible accidents. Ask about the patient's elimination needs professionally, quietly, and allow adequate privacy to avoid further embarrassment.

Before assisting patients to the bathroom, you must first assess their ability to walk. Is the patient dizzy or confused? Is the patient taking medications? Has the patient been walking in the room? Check patients' chart to see if they have bathroom privileges and whether their fluid intake and output (*I & O*) are being measured and recorded. Before escorting patients to the bathroom, make sure they are covered with a robe or sheet and have slippers or shoes on their feet. Orient them to the bathroom, explain the use of a call light if available, and tell them you will wait outside the door. If no call light is available, check on the patient frequently. If patients are on I & O, their urine should be collected in a specimen cup, measured, and recorded before disposal. In some instances, it may be necessary to send the urine back to the nursing unit with the patient for laboratory analysis.

After using the bathroom, patients may need assistance washing their hands. Accompany patients back to their stretchers or wheelchairs, and check the bathroom to make sure it is clean.

BEDPANS

A patient not permitted or able to walk to the bathroom must use a bedpan to defecate. Females also use bedpans to urinate, whereas males use urinals. Bedpans are very uncomfortable for many patients, so help them obtain the most comfortable position possible. If patients are completely immobile or have limited use of their legs, two people should assist them with their bedpan placement.

There are two types of bedpans: regular (Fig. 6-15, *A*) and fracture (Fig. 6-15, *B*). The fracture pan is smaller than a regular pan and is shallow at one end, so it slips easily under the patient.

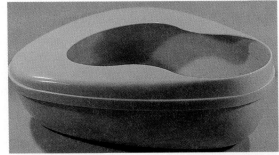 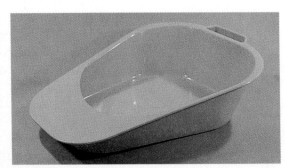

FIG. 6-15 **A,** Regular bedpan. **B,** Fracture bedpan.

PROCEDURE 6-7
ASSISTING PATIENTS WITH BEDPANS

1. Wash your hands and put on a clean pair of gloves.
2. Close the drapes or door to provide privacy.
3. To prevent muscle strain, elevate the head of the bed or cart approximately 30°. If patients are on x-ray tables, position pillows or an angle sponge behind their back to promote comfort.
4. Ask patients to bend their knees and put their feet flat on the bed; then ask patients to raise their hips. Assist patients by placing your hand under the small of their back.
5. With your other hand, slide the bedpan under the patient with the open end toward the patient's feet.
6. Cover the patient with a sheet. Make sure the siderails are up, and ask the patient to call you when finished. Remain outside the door or curtain so that you can respond immediately.
7. Provide toilet tissue for the patient, as well as a wet washcloth to clean the patient's hands afterward.
8. Wearing disposable gloves, remove the bedpan from underneath the patient and dispose of its contents in the toilet.
9. Remove and dispose of your gloves properly, and wash your hands.
10. Record the urine output or bowel elimination in the patient's chart if necessary.

Although most institutions use disposable bedpans and urinals, some hospitals still use metal ones. After sterilization, metal bedpans and urinals are often wrapped in paper and stored with other clean items. When using metal bedpans, hold them under warm, running water and dry them before offering them to patients. Warmed pans help patients relax, which promotes elimination. Procedure 6-7 describes the procedure for helping patients with bedpans.

You may need to assist patients with wiping after they have eliminated. Have a warm, wet washcloth and a dry towel ready. Wear clean gloves. Ask patients to elevate their hips or roll to their side so that you can remove their bedpans. Slide the bedpan *gently* out from under the patient to avoid spilling the contents. Set the bedpan aside, and assist with wiping if needed. Use the warm washcloth, and gently wipe from front to back to prevent feces from entering the urethras or vaginas of female patients. Gently pat the area dry with a dry towel. Help the patient obtain a comfortable position. Measure the amount of urine and assess the stool (if required), empty the bedpan contents into the toilet, and rinse the bedpan

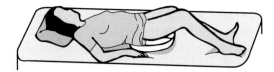

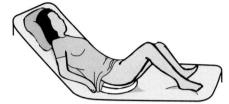

FIG. 6-16 Elevate the patient's head for comfort.

thoroughly (even if it is a disposable bedpan). Dispose of the bedpan properly, or place it in the dirty utility room for cleaning and resterilization. Remove your gloves and wash your hands.

If patients are unable to lift their hips for you so that you can position the bedpan, lower the head of the bed or cart flat, and help patients roll onto their sides away from you. The siderail opposite you should be up. If the patient is lying on the x-ray table, another person should stand on the opposite side of the table to prevent the patient from falling. Place the bedpan firmly against the patient's buttocks, and hold it there with one hand. With your other hand on the patient's hip, guide the patient onto the back and bedpan.

Raise the head of the bed or cart 30°, and make sure the patient is comfortable (Fig. 6-16). Raise the other siderail, and maintain privacy. To remove the bedpan follow the same procedure for rolling patients onto their sides. Help the patient with hygiene.

URINALS

A male patient not permitted or able to walk to the bathroom may use a urinal. Urinals can be metal or disposable. Disposable urinals are usually marked in cubic centimeters (cc) for the measurement of urine output (Fig. 6-17). Male patients can use the urinals while lying supine, on their sides, or in the Fowler's (semisitting) position.

If a male patient cannot put the urinal in the correct position himself, don clean gloves, spread his legs, and place the urinal between them. Place the patient's penis into the urinal. Hold the handle of the urinal with one hand, and use your other hand to cover the patient with the sheet. When the patient is finished urinating, remove the urinal, empty it, and dispose of it properly. Remove your gloves and wash your hands.

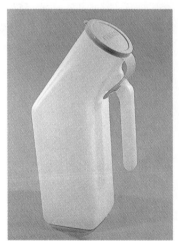

FIG. 6-17
Disposable urinal.

SUMMARY

To provide the best possible care, all patients must be properly prepared for imaging procedures in both ambulatory and inpatient settings. Preparation should consider all aspects of patients' individual physical and psychologic needs. Remember that a patient's most basic needs must be given highest priority. Patients must be protected in safe, comfortable, and private environments. To protect you from potential back injury and provide a safe environment for patients, always apply the principles of good body mechanics when moving patients to or from radiographic tables. Assess vital signs accurately using medical aseptic technique, and document them appropriately for future reference.

STUDY QUESTIONS

1. Compare the patient care needs of ambulatory patients with those of inpatients.
2. List the levels of Maslow's hierarchy of needs. For each level, give an example of how the health care environment or an illness may pose a threat to meeting that level's needs.
3. Describe the six basic components of recording information in a patient's medical record.
4. Specify normal values for the following vital signs:
   A. Temperature
   B. Pulse
   C. Respirations
   D. Blood pressure
5. Name three sites on the body where you may take a pulse measurement.
6. Briefly explain the three principles of good body mechanics and how they apply to an imaging department.
7. Describe three types of patient transfer from a wheelchair or a stretcher.

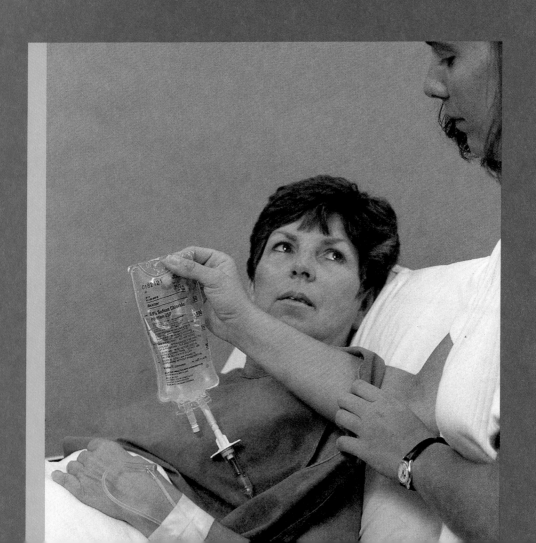

Tubes, Catheters, and Vascular Access Lines

Key Terms

Contents

INTRAVENOUS ACCESS LINES
  FLOW CONTROL DEVICES
  TROUBLESHOOTING IV ACCESS LINES
  CARE OF CENTRAL VASCULAR ACCESS LINES
  SALINE/HEPARIN LOCKS
  SWAN-GANZ CATHETERS
  INFUSION PORTS
TUBES
  NASOGASTRIC TUBES
  GASTRIC TUBES
  FEEDING TUBES
  CHEST TUBES
URINARY SYSTEM CATHETERS AND TUBES
  URINARY CATHETERS
  NEPHROSTOMY TUBES
ABSCESS DRAINAGE TUBES

Objectives

AFTER COMPLETING THIS CHAPTER, THE STUDENT WILL BE ABLE TO:

1. List four reasons a patient may have an IV line in place, and describe the way to maintain patency of the IV.
2. Differentiate between a central and a peripheral vascular access line.

3. Explain the reasons for placement of a gastric or gastrostomy tube and the precautions to take when performing an examination on a patient who has one of these tubes.
4. Describe the responsibility of the technologist to a patient with a urinary catheter.
5. Demonstrate the way to correctly clamp the catheter of a patient receiving continuous irrigation.
6. Explain the technologist's responsibilities to a patient who has a chest tube.

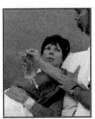 PATIENTS MAY HAVE A VARIETY OF LINES, tubes, and catheters for diagnoses or treatments of conditions affecting the respiratory, urinary, gastrointestinal, or cardiovascular system. You should be familiar with access lines and drainage devices, and use caution when moving or positioning patients who have them in place. Certain lines and tubes, such as nephrostomy tubes, allow access to body systems that are normally sterile, so surgical aseptic techniques must be used to prevent infection. Most of the lines and tubes discussed in this chapter are visible on plain radiographs of the chest or abdomen.

INTRAVENOUS ACCESS LINES

Intravenous access lines (**IVs**) are used for a variety of reasons, which include providing patients with fluids and electrolytes, medications, nutrition, blood products, or chemotherapy. Access lines must remain patent (open) and free from infection.

The most common causes for loss of patency in IV lines are patient movement and improper IV solution height. These problems are especially prevalent in the imaging department. Unless the IV bag is positioned at an appropriate height above the IV site (45 to 60 cm [18 to 24 inches]), the solution may not infuse and the access line may become obstructed by clotting.

When walking patients to the bathroom, use an IV pole to maintain the height of the IV fluid container. You should not carry or lay down the bag. If a patient is on a cart, make sure that the IV pole is high enough to ensure infusion, especially if the patient is sitting. This position exerts more pressure on the vein and may prevent adequate flow of the solution.

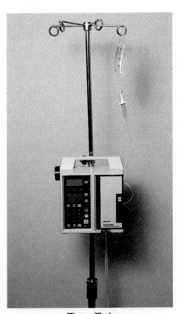

FIG. 7-1
Electronic infusion pump.

FLOW CONTROL DEVICES

Infusion pumps electronically maintain a set flow rate of medication or IV fluid through the vascular access line (Fig. 7-1). This type of medication or fluid delivery is critical for patients who have fluid imbalances or need certain medications or parenteral nutrition. The pump can be operated by batteries during transport or when needed; however, it should be plugged in whenever possible to prevent the batteries from wearing down.

ALERT! If the pump is not plugged in and the batteries fail, the pump usually shuts off and infusion stops. If the infusion does not continue, the IV site will become occluded in 5 minutes or less. If occlusion occurs, contact a nurse in the department immediately.

Most pumps are equipped with controls that regulate the rate and volume of fluid delivered and measure the total volume of fluid infused. These controls are set according to a physician's orders and should not be altered unless you have obtained permission from either the patient's physician or nurse. Built-in alarms signal problems with access lines that may affect infusion. Problems include air in the lines, occlusion, and low batteries, as well as infusion of too little liquid. Know these alarms, and if you have been trained to do so, correct any problems before access lines become occluded. If a problem arises and you have not been trained to operate the pump, call the radiology nurse or patient's nurse from the floor for assistance.

ALERT! If the patient's gown must be changed while in the department and the IV fluid is being infused by a pump, stop the pump. Close the roller clamp on the IV tubing and disengage the tubing from the pump. Closing the tubing roller clamp is very important because when tubing is disengaged from a pump and is completely open, fluid will infuse rapidly and the patient could receive a large infusion of fluid. This could result in a fluid overload, which is particularly dangerous in certain cardiovascular, kidney, and neurologic disorders. Procedure 7-1 describes the steps for changing the patient's gown over an IV.

TROUBLESHOOTING IV ACCESS LINES

Roller clamps also control infusion rates and should not be used to turn off an IV when using an access line for injecting medications and contrast agents. The intravenous flow rate can be affected by the solution height, the size of the IV needle or catheter, a knot or kink in the tubing, and the position of the patient's extremity. A patent needle or catheter has no clots at its end, and its tip is not

PROCEDURE 7-1
CHANGING A PATIENT'S GOWN OVER AN IV

1. Wash your hands and don clean disposable gloves.
2. Untie the patient's soiled gown.
3. Place a clean gown over the patient.
4. Take the patient's unaffected arm out of the dirty gown sleeve, keeping the patient covered.
5. Take the arm with the IV out of the sleeve slowly, taking care not to pull on the tubing or IV site.
6. Pass the IV bag through the sleeve from outside to inside and then through the clean gown sleeve from inside to outside. Place the IV bag back on the stand.
7. Help the patient slide the arm with the IV through the clean gown sleeve. Make sure the tubing is pulled through completely and not caught inside the gown.
8. Remove the soiled gown by pulling it out from under the clean gown from top to bottom. Tie the clean gown.
9. Reset the IV infusion at the correct rate.
10. Dispose of the soiled gown properly. Remove gloves and wash your hands.

against the vein wall. If a problem is suspected, a technologist can assess patency by momentarily lowering the IV bag below the insertion site and checking for a backflow of blood into the tubing. If no blood returns and fluid is not dripping in the drip chamber, there may be a clot in the catheter tip.

If the insertion site appears red or swollen and is painful and cool to the touch, there may be an infiltration of fluid into the tissues. Infiltration occurs when the catheter or needle is dislodged from the vein and fluid flows into (infiltrates) the surrounding tissue. Stop the IV, and remove the needle immediately to prevent phlebitis (inflammation of the vein) or infection. If infiltration occurs, elevate the extremity to promote venous drainage and help decrease edema and apply a warm compress (a towel or washcloth) to the affected area for 20 minutes to increase circulation and reduce pain and edema. Certain medications infiltrating into tissues, such as iodinated contrast agents added to the solution or injected through the IV access line, may cause skin sloughing (surrounding tissue dying and falling off).

An IV may be infusing via a peripheral vein with an over-the-needle catheter or through a central line. Over-the-needle catheters have a relatively low complication rate when properly maintained.

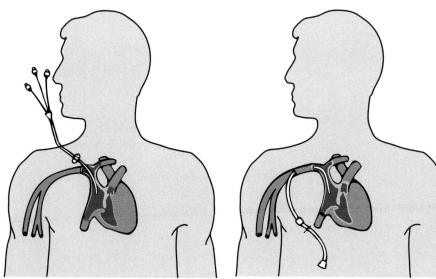

FIG. 7-2 Triple-lumen central venous catheter.

FIG. 7-3 Hickman catheter placement.

Their versatility allows patients to receive treatments in a variety of health care settings.

CARE OF CENTRAL VASCULAR ACCESS LINES

Central lines are single-lumen or multilumen catheters inserted by the physician into a peripheral or central vein. They are used for pressure monitoring; administering medication, total parenteral nutrition (TPN), and blood or blood products; chemotherapy; obtaining blood specimens; or establishing long-term venous access. Incompatible solutions may be infused simultaneously through separate lumens of a multilumen catheter. After insertion and before fluid infusion, catheter placement must be verified by fluoroscopy or radiography. The catheter may be inserted into the subclavian, jugular, or femoral vein for short-term use (with a dual- or triple-lumen catheter), (Fig. 7-2) or the superior vena cava at the junction of the right atrium for long-term use. Different catheters may be used, such as the Hickman, Groshong, or Raff single-, double-, or triple-lumen catheters (Fig. 7-3).

An occlusive sterile dressing should be placed over the insertion site of the central line. Notify the patient's nurse or radiology nurse if the dressing is not in place or secure. See Procedure 7-2 for the steps to flush central lines. Perform this procedure only if it is in your job description or institutional policy.

SHORT-TERM USE (SUBCLAVIAN)

1. Before injection, cleanse a Luer-Lok injection cap with povidone (Betadine). Assess blood return by gently aspirating with a saline-filled syringe.
2. After each use, flush the lumen with 5 ml normal bacteriostatic saline and 2.5 ml heparin (100 U/ml) or according to institutional policy.

LONG-TERM USE (HICKMAN, QUINTON, RAAF)

1. Before injection, cleanse a Luer-Lok injection cap with povidone (Betadine). Assess blood return by gently aspirating with a saline-filled syringe.
2. After each use, flush the lumen with 5 ml normal bacteriostatic saline and 2.5 ml heparin (100 U/ml).

LONG-TERM USE (GROSHONG)

1. Before use, cleanse a Luer-Lok injection cap with povidone (Betadine). Assess blood return by gently aspirating with a saline-filled syringe.
2. After each use, flush the lumen with 5 ml normal bacteriostatic saline. Use force when flushing. (Heparin not required to maintain patency.)

SALINE/HEPARIN LOCKS

A **saline** or **heparin lock** is a special needle with a rubber stopper cap on the end. The saline or heparin lock is placed in the patient's vein and provides intermittent venous access for the administration of medications or fluids or for blood drawing. This device is cost effective for patients who do not require continuous IV fluid therapy and reduces the number of needle sticks the patient receives. Iodinated contrast agents should be injected through these devices when possible to further decrease unnecessary needle sticks.

Flush the lock with heparin or saline according to your institution's policy. Cleanse a saline lock with an alcohol swab before each use. After each use, flush it with 2 to 3 ml of bacteriostatic normal saline. A heparin lock must be flushed with 2 to 3 ml of bacteriostatic normal saline before use and 2.5 ml of heparin (100 U/ml) after use. See Procedures 7-3 and 7-4 for the steps for using a saline and heparin lock.

SWAN-GANZ CATHETERS

Pulmonary artery pressure (PAP) and pulmonary capillary wedge pressure (PCWP) can be measured with a special balloon-tipped

PROCEDURE 7-3
USING A SALINE LOCK

1. Cleanse the lock before each use with an alcohol swab.
2. Fill the syringe with 3 ml bacteriostatic saline, and gently insert the needle into the syringe's hub.
3. Pull back gently to check for blood return in the lock (flashback).
4. If no blood returns, gently attempt to inject a small amount of saline. If you feel resistance, stop and use another site.

ALERT! Do not attempt to force saline through the needle if you feel resistance. The end of the needle may be clotted, and you could force a clot into the bloodstream.

5. If saline flushes easily, proceed with the injection.
6. After injecting the medication or contrast, flush the saline lock with 2 to 3 ml of bacteriostatic saline.

PROCEDURE 7-4
USING A HEPARIN LOCK

1. Cleanse the lock before each use with an alcohol swab.
2. Fill the syringe with 3 ml of bacteriostatic saline, and gently insert the needle into the syringe's hub.
3. Pull back gently to check for blood flashback.
4. If no blood returns, gently attempt to inject a small amount of saline. If you feel resistance, stop and use another site.

ALERT! Do not attempt to force saline through the needle if you feel resistance. The end of the needle may be clotted, and you could force a clot into the bloodstream.

5. If saline flushes easily, proceed with the injection.
6. After the injection, first flush with 2 to 3 ml of bacteriostatic normal saline and then flush with 2.5 ml heparin (100 U/ml) or according to institutional policy.

catheter called a *Swan-Ganz catheter* (Fig. 7-4, *A*). The Swan-Ganz catheter is usually inserted through the subclavian vein and advanced into the right atrium. The balloon is inflated and floated into the pulmonary artery. The balloon is then deflated and is reinflated only when needed to obtain a pressure. The external end of the catheter is connected to a continuous flush system to maintain patency of the catheter. A chest radiograph is used to verify its position after placement or to check the status of the balloon. Except when pressures are being taken, the balloon is deflated and floats freely in the pulmonary artery (Fig. 7-4, *B*).

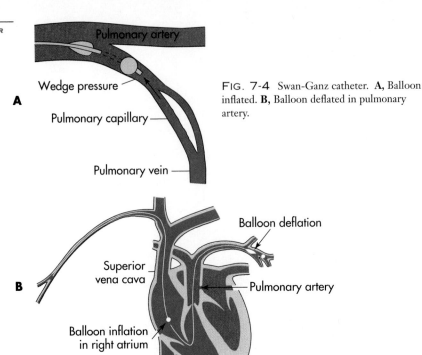

FIG. 7-4 Swan-Ganz catheter. **A,** Balloon inflated. **B,** Balloon deflated in pulmonary artery.

INFUSION PORTS

An implantable **infusion port** is a self-sealing injection port within a plastic or metal case. It is connected to a venous catheter (Fig. 7-5) and implanted by a physician with the patient under local anesthesia in the operating room. The catheter is inserted through the skin into a large vein in the chest. The catheter tip advances into the right atrium. The other end of the catheter tunnels under the skin, usually near the shoulder. The port is placed under the skin through an incision and attached to the catheter. Once the incision is closed, the entire device is under the skin (Fig. 7-6).

The port can be easily palpated under the skin, so its location can be determined for needle access. Specially designed needles such as Huber needles (Fig. 7-7) are used to access the port. Implantable infusion ports may be used for continuous infusions of fluids, blood products, medications, chemotherapy, and parenteral nutrition. They are designed for long-term use and must be heparinized to maintain patency.

Only specially trained personnel should attempt to access infusion ports. The two most common complications are infection and clotting.

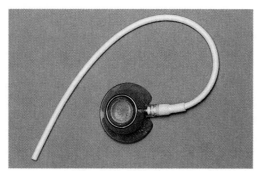

FIG. 7-5 Infusion port.

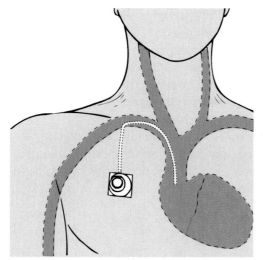

FIG. 7-6 Placement of infusion port.

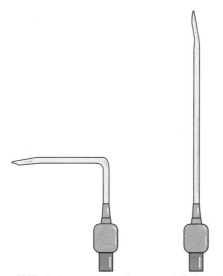

FIG. 7-7 Huber needles used to access infusion port.

TUBES

NASOGASTRIC TUBES

A **nasogastric (NG) tube** is a common type of **gastric tube**. An NG tube is placed through the nose, down the esophagus, and into the stomach. The NG tube has a hollow lumen for removing gastric secretions and gas from the stomach (which is referred to as *decompression*) and introducing liquids into the stomach. The NG tube is used postsurgically to prevent distention of the stomach and vomiting resulting from reduced stomach peristalsis. A reduction in stomach peristalsis results from general anesthesia, manipulation of the viscera during surgery, or obstruction of the operative site by edema. When used for decompression, the NG tube is usually connected to an intermittent- or a low-suction device. The most common NG tubes for decompression include the single-lumen Levin tube, which has several holes near the tip, and the double-lumen Salem sump tube. One lumen in the Salem sump tube is used for removal of gastric contents, and the other is used as an air vent for gas decompression (Fig. 7-8).

If the tube is inserted in the radiology department, the technologist may be responsible for gathering supplies and assisting the radiologist (Procedure 7-5). Because an NG tube can be very uncomfortable for the patient, make sure no tension is on the tube.

GASTRIC TUBES

Some gastrointestinal tubes are used to decompress the intestinal tract rather than the stomach. The Miller-Abbott tube is a double-

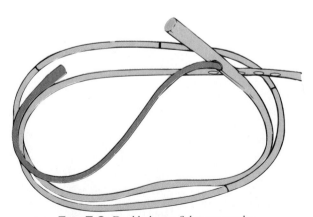

FIG. 7-8 Double-lumen Salem sump tube.

ASSISTING WITH THE INSERTION OF A NASOGASTRIC TUBE

SUPPLIES NEEDED:

- NG tube (large bore: 14 to 18 F, small bore: 8 to 12 F)
- Water-soluble lubricant
- 60 ml catheter-tip syringe
- Glass of water with straw, emesis basin, tissues, tongue blade
- Clean gloves
- Adhesive tape
- Safety pin

1. Explain the procedure to the patient and the reason it is being performed. The procedure is uncomfortable and may be frightening to patients. Reassure and support patients to gain their confidence and ensure their cooperation.
2. Wash your hands. Assemble all equipment.
3. Assist the patient into the Fowler or sitting position on the table.
4. Place a towel over the patient's shoulders to avoid soiling the gown. Give tissues to the patient because the procedure often produces tearing.
5. The radiologist or nurse determines the length of tube to be inserted by measuring the distance from the tip of the nose to the earlobe to the xiphoid process.
6. Wearing clean gloves, the radiologist or nurse lubricates the end of the tube (10 to 20 cm).
7. Tell the patient that the insertion will begin, and explain that frequent sips of water will be given or the patient will be asked to swallow to assist passage of the tube.
8. As the tube is passed through the nares to the back of the throat, the patient may gag or vomit. Make sure that the emesis basin and tissues are available.
9. After the tube has passed through the nasopharynx, allow the patient to rest for a moment.
10. As the tube is advancing, the patient should swallow small sips of water or swallow frequently.
11. When the tube is in place, you may check its placement fluoroscopically or by injecting 10 to 20 ml of air into the tube and auscultating with a stethoscope over the stomach. Air entering the stomach creates a whooshing sound and confirms correct tube placement. The clinician may also aspirate to check for gastric contents. Nothing should be put through an NG tube without first varifying correct placement, regardless of whether the tube was just inserted or has been in place for a significant amount of time.

ALERT! If at any time during the procedure the patient becomes cyanotic, the tube may be in the trachea or coiled or kinked in the back of the mouth. Check inside the mouth with a tongue blade, and gently pull back on the tubing. Allow the patient to rest before proceeding, or administer oxygen as needed.

12. The tube should be secured to the nose with tape. The distal end may be connected to suction or plugged after use and pinned to the patient's gown.
13. Reassure and comfort the patient after the procedure.
14. Dispose of the equipment, remove your gloves, and wash your hands.
15. Record the type of tube used and the patient's tolerance of the procedure in the patient's chart.

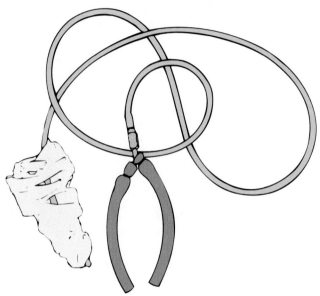

FIG. 7-9 Miller-Abbott double-lumen decompression tube.

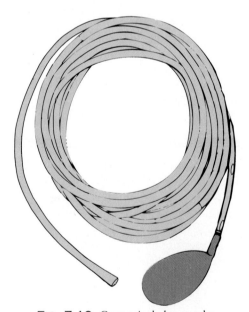

FIG. 7-10 Cantor single-lumen tube.

lumen tube (Fig. 7-9). One lumen is for a balloon, and the other has openings to permit drainage. The balloon is filled with 5 to 9 ml of mercury, water, or air to simulate a bolus of food, thereby stimulating peristalsis in the intestine. Peristalsis advances the tube along the intestinal tract, or in the absence of peristalsis, the weight of the mercury in the balloon carries it forward.

The catheter passes through the stomach with the balloon deflated. The external end of the tube contains two openings, one for drainage (marked *suction*) and one for balloon inflation. The balloon outlet should be clearly marked so that it is not accidently used improperly.

The Cantor tube is a single-lumen tube with one opening for drainage (Fig. 7-10). Mercury is injected into the balloon with a needle and syringe (which occurs before the tube is inserted). The needle opening is small enough to prevent the globules of mercury from escaping.

FEEDING TUBES

NASOGASTRIC TUBES

Some feeding tubes are small-bore (8 to 12 F) NG tubes used to provide nutrition to patients who are unable to feed themselves, will not feed themselves, or who cannot maintain adequate oral nutrition (such as patients with cancer, sepsis, or trauma, or patients who are comatose).

Tube (enteral) feeding is preferred over parenteral nutrition because it allows the body to better use nutrients, is safer for the patient, and is less expensive. Patients whose gastrointestinal systems cannot digest and absorb nutrients are not candidates for tube feedings. They must receive nutrients by the total parenteral nutrition (TPN) method.

Tube feedings use a special pump that is similar to an IV infusion pump. This pump should be turned off any time a patient must be placed in a supine position to avoid aspiration of gastric contents. In many institutions a patient is not allowed to be transported off the unit while the pump is running. If you are unsure whether the pump is running or the way to position a patient with a tube feeding, consult the patient's nurse or physician.

Patients with NG or feeding tubes should not eat or drink anything unless it has been specifically ordered. If you must instill barium through an NG or a feeding tube, make sure the tube is placed correctly, and put the patient in a semi-Fowler's position to prevent aspiration.

PERCUTANEOUS ENDOSCOPIC GASTROSTOMY TUBES

The percutaneous endoscopic gastrostomy (PEG) tube is a safer, more rapid method to provide nutrition for patients unable to swallow for a long period of time. Gastrostomy creates an opening into the abdomen by insertion of a tube through the stomach wall. While the patient is under local or general anesthesia, a small incision is made in the skin and a cannula is advanced through to the gastric wall while being observed through a gastroscope. A long silk suture passes through the cannula, is grasped by the gastroscope, and is pulled up through the patient's mouth. A special mushroom catheter, or jejunostomy tube, is attached to the thread and pulled retrograde through the esophagus and stomach and out the abdominal wall. Internal and external fixation devices hold the catheter in place.

If barium is given through the PEG tube, the patient's head must be elevated during the procedure and at least 30 min afterward to prevent regurgitation and aspiration.

CHEST TUBES

Chest tubes promote fluid drainage after chest or lung surgery and prevent air or fluid from entering the pleural space. If the patient

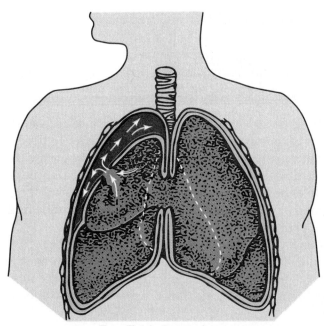

FIG. 7-11 Pneumothorax.

PROCEDURE 7-7

FEMALE URINARY CATHETERIZATION WITH AN INDWELLING CATHETER

Perform steps 1 through 12 of the procedure for using a straight catheter (Procedure 7-6).

13. Check the catheter balloon by inserting the syringe tip through the valve of the intake lumen and injecting sterile fluid until the balloon inflates. (This procedure checks the strength of the balloon.) Aspirate all of the fluid out of the balloon with the syringe. Leave the syringe attached to the valve.

14. Perform steps 13 through 21 of Procedure 7-6.

15. While holding the patient's meatus with the thumb and little finger of your nondominant hand, use an indwelling (Foley) catheter to slowly inject the amount of solution designated for the size of the balloon being used.

If the patient complains of sudden pain, aspirate the fluid and advance the catheter farther.

16. After fully inflating the balloon, release the catheter with your nondominant hand and pull gently to feel resistance.

17. Attach the end of the catheter to the collecting tube of the drainage bag.

18. Tape the catheter to the patient's inner thigh with a strip of nonallergenic tape. Allow for some slack in the tubing so that thigh movements do not pull on the catheter.

19. Be sure that the tubing is free from obstructions, kinking, or tension. Position the drainage bag on the lower side of bed or cart (on the side that has the leg with tubing).

20. Dispose of equipment, drapes, and urine in the proper receptacles.

21. Help the patient obtain a comfortable position. Wash and dry the perineal area as needed.

22. Warn the patient not to pull or put unnecessary tension on the tubing when changing positions.

23. Remove your gloves and wash your hands.

24. Record the results of the procedure in the patient's chart, including the size of the catheter, the character and amount of urine, and the patient's tolerance of the procedure.

ALERT! If the catheter is mistakenly introduced into the patient's vagina (as evidenced by absence of urine flow or leaking of instilled solution), leave it in place because it provides a landmark for correct placement of the catheter into the urethra. Open a new sterile catheter and place it in the urethra (which is immediately anterior to the vagina). Remove the misplaced catheter.

PROCEDURE 7-8
MALE CATHETERIZATION WITH A STRAIGHT CATHETER

1. Assist the patient into the supine position with his thighs slightly abducted.
2. Open the catheterization kit and establish a sterile field. Put on sterile gloves and follow steps 11 through 13 of Procedure 7-6.
3. Apply a drape over the thighs just below the penis. Pick up the fenestrated sterile drape, allow it to unfold, and drape it over the penis, allowing the fenestrated slit to rest over the penis.
4. Cleanse the urethral meatus. (For uncircumcised males, retract the foreskin with your nondominant hand.)
5. Grasp the penis shaft just below the glans. Retract the urethral meatus between your thumb and forefinger. Keep your nondominant hand in this position throughout the procedure.
6. With your dominant hand, pick up a cotton ball with forceps and clean the penis. Move it in a circular motion from the meatus down to the base of the glans. Repeat this cleansing 2 more times, using a clean cotton ball each time.
7. Pick up the catheter with your gloved, dominant hand 7 to 10 cm (3 to 4 inches) from the catheter tip.
8. Lift the penis to a position perpendicular to the patient's body, and apply light traction.
9. Ask the patient to bear down as if voiding and slowly insert the catheter through the meatus.
10. Advance the catheter 15 to 22 cm (7 to 9 inches) in adults and 5 to 8 cm (2 to 3 inches) in young children or until urine flows out the catheter's end or into the collection bag. If you feel resistance, withdraw the catheter. Do not force it through the urethra, and ask for assistance from a physician or nurse. When urine appears, advance the catheter another 5 cm (2 inches).
11. Lower the penis, and hold the catheter securely in your nondominant hand. If using a straight catheter, place the end of the catheter in the urine tray receptacle. Allow the bladder to empty.
12. Remove the straight catheter.
13. Dispose of equipment and urine in the proper receptacles. Remove your gloves and wash your hands.
14. Record the results of the procedure in the patient's chart, including the size of the catheter, the character and amount of urine, and the patient's tolerance of the procedure.

PROCEDURE 7-9
MALE CATHETERIZATION WITH AN INDWELLING CATHETERS

Perform steps 1 through 10 of the procedure for using a straight catheter (Procedure 7-8).

11. Inflate the balloon of the indwelling catheter. While holding the catheter in place at the meatus with your non-dominant hand, slowly inject the fluid into the balloon, but do not exceed the designated balloon capacity.
12. If the patient complains of pain, the balloon may be malpositioned in the urethra; aspirate the solution and advance the catheter farther and reinject the solution.
13. Gently pull back on the catheter to determine whether there is resistance.
14. Attach the end of the catheter to the collecting tube of the drainage bag.
15. Tape the catheter to the patient's inner thigh with a strip of nonallergenic tape. Allow slack in the tubing so that thigh movements do not pull on the catheter.
16. Be sure that the tubing is free from obstructions, kinking, or tension. Place the drainage bag at the lower side of the bed or cart on the side with the tubing.
17. Dispose of equipment, drapes, and urine in the proper receptacles.
18. Help the patient to a comfortable position.
19. Warn the patient not to pull or put unnecessary tension on the tubing when changing positions.
20. Remove your gloves and wash your hands.
21. Record the results of the procedure in the patient's chart, including the size of the catheter, the character and amount of urine, and the patient's tolerance of the procedure.

PROCEDURE 7-10
REMOVAL OF AN INDWELLING FOLEY CATHETER

1. Wash your hands and don clean disposable gloves.
2. Position the patient in the supine position.
3. Place a waterproof pad between female patients' thighs or over male patients' thighs.
4. Obtain a sterile urine specimen if needed.
5. Insert the hub of the syringe into the inflate valve. Aspirate the entire amount of fluid used to inflate the balloon. (Note the balloon capacity.)
6. Pull the catheter out slowly and smoothly. Stop if resistance is met; the balloon may still be partially inflated.)
7. Measure and empty the contents of the collection bag.
8. Dispose of all contaminated supplies.
9. Wash your hands.
10. Document the procedure, time, amount of urine, patient's tolerance of the procedure, and any difficulties encountered in the patient's chart.

leave the bag on the cart or table or hold it above the patient's bladder level when helping the patient walk.

CLAMPING OF URINARY CATHETERS

If a patient has an indwelling catheter and you are performing an IV urogram or are trying to visualize the bladder after injection of contrast media, clamp the catheter distal to the connection between the catheter and collection bag tubing. Use a screw-type clamp or forceps without teeth (to prevent puncturing tubing) to gently clamp the tubing. Make sure no tension is placed on the catheter by the clamp.

If the patient has an indwelling catheter with an irrigation solution running, be very careful to prevent injury to the patient. Catheter irrigation is frequently used after bladder surgery to remove blood clots that may have formed in the bladder and maintain the patency of the catheter. The collection bags are usually larger so that they can accommodate more fluid, especially during continuous irrigation.

ALERT! Make sure the collection bag is supported so that no tension is placed on the catheter from the weight of the fluid in the bag. Check the bag frequently and empty it when it is full to prevent backflow of urine into the catheter or clotting in the catheter.

If you need to empty a full urine collection bag, always record the amount, color, and consistency of the urine (for example, "2000 ml dark-red urine with clots") in the patient's chart. If you are unfamiliar with the way to empty the collection bag, contact the radiology nurse or patient's nurse before proceeding.

A physician's or radiologist's order is required before clamping the catheter tubing of a patient receiving continuous irrigation. Clamp the irrigation solution tubing. (Do not use the roller clamp because this will change the rate of infusion.) Then clamp the tubing to the collection bag. Using this procedure prevents overdistention of the bladder. Proceed with the examination.

After the examination, reverse the procedure by unclamping the tubing to the collection bag first, and then unclamp the tubing from the irrigation solution. This prevents overdistention of the bladder and possible injury.

NEPHROSTOMY TUBES

A percutaneous **nephrostomy tube** is often inserted in patients who have urinary tract obstructions or who are going to have percutaneous lithotripsy for renal stones. The tube may be inserted in surgery with an endoscope or under sterile conditions in the radiology department using fluoroscopy.

With the patient in a prone or semiprone position, a small incision is made through the skin over the kidney region. A needle is inserted into the renal pelvis or calyx, and a wire is passed through the needle into the ureter. The tract is dilated, and a pigtail-style catheter with multiple side holes for drainage (Fig. 7-15) is inserted into the renal pelvis or calyx. The size of the catheter is determined by its intended function. For example, a larger catheter is inserted if the tract will eventually be used for lithotripsy.

When the wire and needle are withdrawn, the catheter assumes a pigtail configuration within the kidney. The catheter is then connected to an external drainage bag and secured by an external fixation device or with sutures. Do not put any tension on the catheter when moving or positioning the patient. If the catheter disconnects or the dressing saturates, notify the nurse or radiologist.

ABSCESS DRAINAGE TUBES

An **abscess** is an abnormal collection of pus that can occur in any organ or part of the body. A patient with an abscess may have a drainage tube (Fig. 7-16) so be careful not to disconnect or dislodge the catheter when moving or positioning the patient. An abscess can be very painful, and the patient usually has a fever.

Monitor patients with abscess drainage tubes for signs of sepsis or systemic infection, such as chilling, tachycardia, high fever, or confusion. Most patients with abscesses receive antibiotic therapy, which is critical for preventing further infection.

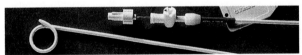

FIG. 7-15 Nephrostomy tube. (Courtesy Medi-tech/Boston Scientific Corp.)

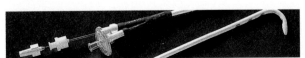

FIG. 7-16 Van Sonnenberg drainage tube. (Courtesy Medi-tech/Boston Scientific Corp.)

SUMMARY

As an imaging professional, you will work with patients who have a variety of vascular access devices, drainage tubes, and catheters. In some instances, you may be involved in interventional procedures that include the insertion of stents or catheters. You must be knowledgeable about and skilled with performing a variety of radiographic procedures on patients with IV access lines, gastric tubes, chest tubes, and urinary catheters. You must be able to differentiate among the uses and radiographic appearances of various access lines and tubes. Life-threatening complications may occur if lines, tubes, or catheters are not cared for properly.

STUDY QUESTIONS

1. Why should you close the roller clamp on an IV when disconnecting the IV tubing from an infusion pump?
2. How does a central vascular access line differ from a peripheral IV access line?
3. What steps must be taken to ensure patency of a vascular access line?
4. In which position should patients be placed before you instill barium sulfate through their NG tubes?
5. How do NG tubes differ from tubes that decompress gas in the intestines?
6. What is the purpose of a chest tube?
7. Describe the procedure for clamping the urinary catheter of a patient who is receiving continuous bladder irrigation.
8. Describe the way to remove a urinary catheter after a cystogram.

Eight

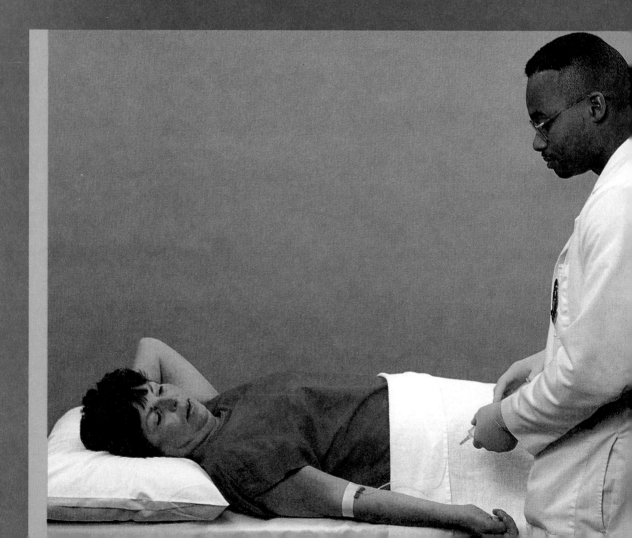

Medication Administration

Key Terms

Contents

Objectives

AFTER COMPLETING THIS CHAPTER, THE STUDENT WILL BE ABLE TO:

1. List the components of a medication order.
2. List the *five rights* of medication administration.
3. Describe the factors affecting drug administration.
4. Differentiate among the methods of medication administration, and explain the way the route of administration can be determined.
5. Identify and define common abbreviations used in medication administration.
6. List resources available for drug information.
7. Demonstrate the procedure for drawing medication from a vial and an ampule.
8. Differentiate among the classifications and uses of various drugs used in the radiology department.
9. Describe sites that are commonly used for a venipuncture.
10. Demonstrate several methods for locating veins that are hard to find.
11. Demonstrate the procedure used for a venipuncture.
12. List the symptoms of infiltration.
13. Describe the various needles that may be used for a venipuncture.
14. Identify which universal precautions should be taken by a person performing a venipuncture.
15. Differentiate between the uses and radiographic appearances of positive and negative contrast agents.
16. List specific agents commonly used as positive and negative contrast materials.
17. Identify the specific types of contrast agents that can be injected into the bloodstream.
18. Compare ionic and nonionic positive contrast agents.

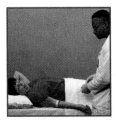 IN THE HEALTH CARE FIELD THE TERMS *medications* and *drugs* are often used synonymously. In most states, medications must be prescribed by physicians or dentists. A technologist, however, may administer various medications for radiographic procedures. These include medications for sedation and pain management, contrast media, and emergency drugs for contrast reactions.

Because of risks to the patient and legal liabilities, technologists must follow state regulations and hospital policies when administering any medication. Administering drugs accurately and safely is an important responsibility and should not be taken lightly. Any medication has the potential to be harmful if it is not administered properly.

Technologists should be familiar with the frequently used drugs in their departments. Know the names of drugs, goals of drug therapies, dosages, contraindications, and proper administration methods. Be aware of expected and unusual effects produced by certain drugs. Anticipate and be prepared to assist physicians with treatment for any unexpected reactions. Any medication can produce side effects or reactions in certain patients. The technologist, who is often the only health care professional in direct contact with the patient at this time, should notice any signs or symptoms of allergic reactions or side effects. Immediately report these to the physician if they occur.

Several resources that help identify medications, their dosages, uses, and contraindications are available to technologists. The easiest resource to find is usually the medication's package insert, which lists its generic name, trade name, chemical composition, chemical strength, usual dosage, indications, contraindications, and reported side effects. The *Physician's Desk Reference* (PDR), which is published annually, lists drugs alphabetically by their generic names, trade names, and uses. Its index has several sections for cross-referencing drugs by their manufacturers, classifications, and uses.

MEDICATION NOMENCLATURE

A medication may be referred to by its chemical, generic, or trade name. The chemical name represents the exact composition of the drug. These names are often long and difficult to pronounce. In some cases, a drug's chemical and generic names may be the same. **Generic names** are given to medications by their original manufacturers before the medications receive official approval by the federal government's Food and Drug Administration (FDA). Generic names are nonproprietary (specific to the drug but not to the pharmaceutical company manufacturing the drug) and are used before and after FDA approval.

The generic name is always on the medication package, but it may be in lower case letters that are in small print. A drug may also be called by its proprietary name, also known as its brand or **trade name**. The trade name is given by a pharmaceutical company to its own specific product. Generic drugs may be available from a variety of manufacturers and sold under different trade names. For instance, *acetaminophen* is the generic name for an analgesic (painkiller) commonly used in hospitals. This drug is manufactured by a variety of pharmaceutical companies, and its most common trade names are *Tylenol* and *Panadol*. Many drugs have similar trade names, so it is critical to know the exact name and spelling of the drug you are working with in each situation.

MEDICATION ORDERS

Orders for medications can be verbal or written, but both types must be signed by the ordering physician within 24 hr of being ordered. Ask the physician to clarify any order that is not completely understandable. A medication order must include the date the order was written and the drug's name, dosage, route of administration, and frequency of administration. A drug's frequency is how often and at what time a drug is given. Physicians frequently use abbreviations in medication orders (Table 8-1); be sure you know exactly what all abbreviations mean, and ask the physician if you have any doubts.

MEDICATION ADMINISTRATION

For the patient's safety, there are certain steps to follow before giving them any medication or contrast medium (which is also considered a medication). The *five rights* of safe medication administration (box) are the right patient, right drug, right dosage, right time, and right route. You must confirm these five pieces of information before administering a medication. Ask each patient about any known drug allergies and sensitivities before administering any drug. The box on safe drug administration lists other rules.

RIGHT PATIENT

Always verify that you are administering medication to the right patient. Ask patients their full names; do not say patients' names and assume their responses indicate that you are administering to the right patients. If possible, check patients' identification bracelets in

TABLE 8-1

ABBREVIATIONS OF MEDICATION ADMINISTRATION TERMS

a.c.	before meals	oz	ounce
ad lib.	as desired	p	after
b.i.d.	two times a day	p.c.	after meals
c	with	p.o.	by mouth
cc	cubic centimeter	p.r.n.	when necessary
et	and	q	every
G or gm	gram	q.h.	every hour
gtt	drop	q.4 h	every 4 hours
h	hour	q.4 0	every 4 hours
h.s.	at bedtime	q.i.d.	4 times per day
IM	intramuscular	s	without
IV	intravenous	stat	immediately
kg	kilogram	SQ, subq	subcutaneous
lb	pound	t.i.d.	three times per day
mcg	microgram	T, tbsp	tablespoon
mg	milligram	tsp	teaspoon
mL	milliliter	U	unit
OTC	over the counter		

THE *FIVE RIGHTS* OF SAFE MEDICATION ADMINISTRATION

1. *Right* patient
2. *Right* drug
3. *Right* dosage
4. *Right* time
5. *Right* route

addition to asking their names. Do not administer medication if you are unsure of a patient's identity.

RIGHT DRUG

Check the medication name at least 3 times before it is administered. Check once as you remove the medication from the drawer or shelf, a second time as you prepare the medication for administration, and a third time before you actually administer the drug. Remember that the same medication may have a variety of names (chemical, generic, or trade). Never administer a drug that is in an unlabeled container or syringe.

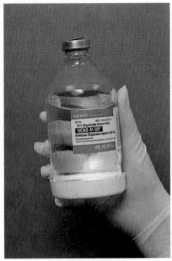

FIG. 8-1

Check the name of the medication, its
strength, and the expiration date.

RULES FOR SAFE DRUG ADMINISTRATION

- Be informed about each drug ordered.
- Use aseptic technique when preparing medications and handling all equipment.
- Respect a patient's right to be informed of the drug's name, purpose, actions, and possible side effects.
- Respect a patient's right to refuse a medication.
- When preparing a medication, always check its name, strength, and expiration date (Fig. 8-1).
- Only administer a medication that you have prepared. You are responsible for the medication you administer, regardless of who has prepared it.
- Before administering medications, ask patients to state their names, and verify they match the names on their identification bracelets.
- Never record that a patient has received a medication before you have actually administered it.
- Record medication immediately after its administration. Also record the patient's response to the drug, any undesired effects, and if the patient refused the medication, the reason it was refused.
- If a medication error is made, a report must be filled out according to institutional policy. The patient's physician must also be notified.
- To be prepared for a serious drug reaction, know where the resuscitation equipment is kept in the department and be familiar with the code procedure of the institution.

RIGHT DOSE

Medications are not always dispensed from the pharmacy or pharmaceutical company in the amount in which they are to be administered. Drug companies bottle contrast agents in standard amounts, however, and it is important to double-check the proper dosage. Pay close attention to decimal points and prefixes (such as milli-, micro-, and centi-) in both the medication order and the packaging.

RIGHT TIME

The physician may give specific instructions about when to administer a medication. Timing is especially important when preparing patients for imaging procedures. Certain drugs may be administered to premedicate patients for procedures. Certain imaging procedures require that the contrast material be administered at a specific time before the procedure begins. Verify the proper medication administration times before beginning a procedure.

RIGHT ROUTE

Medications are available in a variety of forms, including capsules, caplets, elixirs, pills, solutions, suppositories, suspensions, syrup, tablets, and transdermal patches. A medication's form determines its route of administration. In most imaging departments, medications may be ingested, injected, inhaled, or administered rectally in the form of enemas or suppositories.

FACTORS AFFECTING DRUG ADMINISTRATION

Consider the following factors when administering medication to a patient: age; gender; body weight; emotional or psychologic state; time of day; **drug tolerance** (need for increasingly larger doses to achieve the desired response); **drug resistance** (inability to achieve desired response from a drug because of long-term use); liver, renal, and gastrointestinal functioning; and route of drug administration. Age is an important factor, for example, because pediatric and geriatric patients have metabolic systems that respond differently to medications. Gender is also an important factor because in general, males tend to have higher body weights than females, so they may require a different dosage of medication to obtain the same results as a female.

METABOLISM

The liver is the primary site of drug **metabolism** (breakdown of drugs for use in the body). Metabolism transforms drugs into water-soluble substances that can be used by the body and then excreted by the kidneys. Metabolism can also take place in the lungs, kidneys, intestines, and bloodstream.

ABSORPTION

Absorption of a drug can be affected by its chemical composition, an interaction with other drugs or food in the body, body weight and composition, and the route of administration.

ROUTES OF ADMINISTRATION

A drug may be administered **parenterally** (by injection), orally, sublingually, rectally, or topically. The physician selects the route of administration based on the properties of the drug and the desired response time. The parenteral, oral, and sublingual routes are most often used in imaging departments and are the only routes discussed here.

ORAL

The oral route (PO, meaning "per os" or "by mouth") is often the easiest and most desirable route for the patient. Oral medications may be in liquid, tablet, granule, or capsule form. Do not, however, give patients medications by mouth in the following situations:

- The patient is nauseated or vomiting or is likely to feel nauseous or vomit because of the medication's bad taste.
- Digestive juices may interfere with the absorption of the drug, or the drug may irritate the gastric mucosa. (In this situation the medication should be given in an enteric-coated form.)
- The patient is comatose or uncooperative, or there is a danger of aspiration.
- More rapid absorption is needed than can be achieved.

When administering oral medications, begin by washing your hands and verifying that you have the right drug. Do not touch the medication with your hands when preparing it for administration. Place the medication in a medicine cup. When pouring liquids, be sure to pour them from the side of the bottle opposite the label, and wipe the lip of the bottle with a paper towel to ensure the label remains clean and legible.

A patient must be alert and able to swallow well before receiving any oral medications. Place the patient in the most upright position possible to avoid aspiration or choking, and stay with the patient to ensure the medication is swallowed. After the medication has been administered, wash your hands once again and document the medication administration information on the patient's chart.

Absorption by the oral route takes approximately 30 to 45 minutes and depends on the drug administered, any food ingested before or after the medication was given, and any alterations in the patient's digestive process.

PARENTERAL

The parenteral route of drug administration refers to medications given by injection rather than orally (through the digestive system) or rectally. Parenteral routes include intravenous (IV), intramuscular (IM), and subcutaneous (SQ or SC) injections. All types of injections require the use of a needle and syringe and must be performed following proper aseptic technique (see Chapter 5). Universal precautions must be taken at all times when administering medications via a parenteral route. Medications administered parenterally are absorbed into the bloodstream more rapidly than those administered orally.

INTRAVENOUS

A medication given by an IV route is absorbed quickly and leads to a rapid response. Emergency drugs, certain sedative drugs, and some drugs that cannot be absorbed by the digestive system are commonly given intravenously. Because these drugs enter the bloodstream, the technologist must know which to inject quickly and which to inject slowly over a few minutes so that they can elicit the desired response and avoid possible phlebitis (inflammation of the blood vessel). Some medications may be given either intravenously or intramuscularly, such as meperidine (Demerol) and diphenhydramine (Benadryl). Because the medication dose for IV administration is usually much less than for IM, be certain which route the physician has ordered.

INTRAMUSCULAR

Medication administered by the IM route is injected into the deltoid (upper arm), gluteus maximus (posterior hip), or vastus lateralis muscle (lateral aspect of the thigh). Absorption generally takes 15 to 20 minutes, although the time can be decreased by massaging or exercising the muscle site of injection. Generally, larger amounts of up to 3 ml in adults are safely tolerated in larger muscles. Pediatric and geriatric patients, as well as thin adults, can usually only tolerate less than 2 ml of medication without severe discomfort. When performing IM injections, use needles from 1 to 1½ inches in length, with the needle inserted at a right angle (90°) to the muscle (Fig. 8-2).

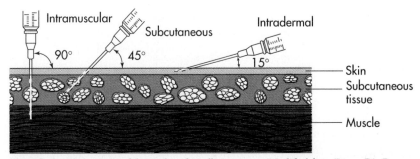

FIG. 8-2 Comparison of the angles of needle insertion. (Modified from Potter PA, Perry AG, *Fundamentals of nursing: concepts, process, and practice*, ed 3, St Louis, 1993, Mosby.)

SUBCUTANEOUS

SQ or SC (under the skin) injections are used for insulin, epinephrine, narcotics, and vaccines. These drugs are water soluble, nonirritating, and nonviscous. The skin only tolerates small amounts of medication (0.5 to 1 ml) without irritation. SQ injections require a 25-gauge needle, that is ⅝ inch in length for adults and ½ inch in length for children. The needle is inserted at a 45° angle to the skin (see Fig. 8-2). SQ tissue is not very vascular, so drugs injected subcutaneously are not absorbed as quickly as those injected by the IM route. An exception is heparin, which is absorbed quickly by both SQ and IM routes.

INTRADERMAL

Intradermal (between layers of skin) injections are rarely used in imaging departments today because skin testing a patient's sensitivity to contrast media has been found to be ineffective. Drug absorption occurs most slowly by this route, and only small amounts of medication (0.01 to 0.1 ml) are used. Needle gauges and lengths are the same as those used for SQ injections, but needles are inserted at a 15° angle to the skin (see Fig. 8-2).

TABLE 8-2

EXAMPLES OF COMMON DRUG CLASSIFICATIONS

CLASSIFICATION	GENERIC NAME	EXAMPLES OF TRADE NAMES
Antiarrhythmic	Propranolol hydrochloride	Inderal, Inderide
	Lidocaine hydrochloride	Lidocaine, Xylocaine
Analgesic	Aspirin	Anacin, Ascripton, Bayer, Bufferin
	Acetaminophen	Tylenol, Panadol
Antibiotic	Penicillin	Amoxicillin, Augmentin
	Cefaclor	Ceclor
Anticoagulant	Crystalline warfarin sodium	Coumadin
	Heparin	Heparin
Antihistamine	Diphenhydramine hydrochloride	Benadryl
Antipyretic	Aspirin	Anacin, Ascripton, Bayer, Bufferin
	Acetaminophen	Tylenol, Panadol
Bronchodilator	Epinephrine	Adrenalin
	Theophylline ethylenediamine	Aminophyllin
Laxative	Bisacodyl	Bisacodyl, Dulcolax, Fleet
Sedative	Sodium thiopental	Pentothal
	Flurazepam hydrochloride	Dalmane, Flurazepam
Vasodilator	Nitroglycerin	Nitro-bid, Nitrocine, Nitrostat
	Verapamil hydrochloride	Isoptin, Verapamil
Vasopressor	Metaraminol bitartrate	Aramine
	Methoxamine hydrochloride	Vasoxyl
	Norepinephrine bitartrate	Levophed Bitartrate

Sublingual (SL) medications are placed under the tongue where they dissolve and are absorbed directly into the bloodstream from the oral mucosa. The medication is not swallowed and does not enter the gastrointestinal (GI) tract or hepatic system. This method of absorption allows a response to occur within seconds. Sublingual drugs may be in tablet (nitroglycerin), spray (also nitroglycerin), capsule (nifedipine [Procardia]), or liquid form.

After administering SL medications, instruct patients to close their mouths and not swallow. Patients should leave the tablet or liquid in place until it has been absorbed.

MEDICATION CLASSIFICATIONS

Medications are typically classified according to a similar, shared characteristic such as their effects on the body (Table 8-2). However, some medications may belong to more than one class. For instance, aspirin may be classified as an analgesic (pain reliever), antipyretic (fever reducer), and antiinflammatory drug.

FREQUENTLY USED MEDICATIONS

Certain medications are regularly used in the radiology department. The specific drugs used at your institution may differ from those used in other institutions, but the drug categories are generally the same.

ALLERGY MEDICATIONS

Antihistamines are frequently used to counteract reactions or allergies. The most common antihistamine, which is diphenhydramine (Benadryl), is used to reduce the itching and discomfort associated with hives. It also has mild sedative and anticholinergic effects (causing drowsiness and dry mouth). Benadryl may be given orally before a procedure in which patients are expected to have an allergic reaction. The usual oral dose is 25 to 50 mg PO. It may be given by the IM or IV route if a patient is having an allergic reaction to a contrast agent. The usual IM or IV dose is 10 to 50 mg; up to 100 mg may be given as needed. The maximum permissible dose in a 24-hr period is 400 mg.

To counteract an acute allergic reaction such as angioedema, shock, or respiratory arrest, epinephrine (Adrenalin) is the drug of choice. It produces bronchodilation by relaxing the nonvascular smooth muscles of the airway and raises blood pressure by constricting peripheral blood vessels. It is administered subcutaneously, intramuscularly, or intravenously. After administration, monitor the patient closely for cardiac arrhythmias or hypertension. The dosage is small (0.2 to 1 ml of 1:1000 solution), and the drug is administered by the physician.

Corticosteroids such as methylprednisolone (Solu-Medrol) and hydrocortisone (Solu-Cortef) may be used when patients with severe allergic reactions do not respond to the previously mentioned treatments. The antiinflammatory components of these drugs prevent or reduce laryngeal and bronchial edema, thus reducing the possibility of respiratory arrest. Solu-Medrol and Solu-Cortef are each packaged in two-compartment vials that have diluents in one compartment and soluble powder in the other; the vial compartments are separated by a rubber stopper. Be familiar with the procedure for mixing this medication *before* the need to do so arises.

NARCOTIC AND NONNARCOTIC ANALGESICS

Analgesics are used to reduce or relieve pain. They may be narcotic or nonnarcotic. Examples of narcotics include morphine, meperidine (Demerol), and codeine. These drugs are **controlled substances**; they have a greater potential for patients to abuse and become dependent on them, so they cannot be dispensed without a prescription. Narcotics must be signed out in a drug book. Any unused portion must be discarded in the presence of a witness, who must also sign the book and verify the disposal. All health care institutions must have policies regarding the proper storage and distribution of controlled substances. Violations of federal mandates (such as the Controlled Substances Act) are punishable by fines, imprisonment, and loss of professional licenses. In the radiology department these drugs are usually limited to use during interventional procedures.

Nonnarcotic analgesics include acetaminophen (Tylenol), aspirin, and ibuprofen (Motrin). Ibuprofen and aspirin may cause GI discomfort unless taken with food or milk. Aspirin can cause GI bleeding when taken in large doses or in conjunction with blood thinners because aspirin also inhibits platelet aggregation (clotting).

ANTIBIOTICS

Antibiotics prevent or destroy bacteria, fungi, or parasites that cause infections in the body. The antibiotic used depends on the organism causing the infection. Antibiotics are generally very effective; however, they do have associated complications, which include the following:

1. Tissue damage
   - Many antibiotics irritate the intestines, causing vomiting, diarrhea, or stomach discomfort.
   - Antibiotics may cause phlebitis when infused intravenously or when they infiltrate tissues.
   - Renal toxicity and ototoxicity (hearing impairment) are the most serious complications of antibiotic administration.
2. Allergies
   - A patient may be mildly hypersensitive to an antibiotic or may have a severe and possibly life-threatening anaphylactic reaction.
3. Superinfection
   - A superinfection is a secondary infection caused by a different organism than the first that occurs as a complication of the first infection.
4. Resistance
   - Patients may develop resistance to certain antibiotics as a result of improper use. For instance, viruses do not respond to antibiotic treatment. However, if an antibiotic is prescribed to treat an upper respiratory virus, the patient may be resistant to the drug when it is later appropriately prescribed to treat an infection. A drug will no longer be therapeutic if a patient has developed a resistance to that drug.

In hospitalized patients who have an IV line in place, antibiotics are administered by IV piggyback (IVPB) into the existing IV line. Therefore piggyback IV lines prevent additional needle punctures. Normally the needle is inserted into the existing tubing using sterile technique. They are usually mixed with dextrose or normal saline in a 50 to 250 ml bag.

ANTIPYRETICS

Antipyretics reduce body temperature. Aspirin and acetaminophen are the most common antipyretics.

ANTIEMETICS

Antiemetics, such as the phenothiazines (Phenergan and Compazine), act on the chemoreceptor trigger zone in the brain to inhibit nausea and vomiting. Antihistamines (such as Benadryl, Vistaril, and Dramamine) are more commonly used to prevent the nausea or vomiting associated with motion sickness. They block histamine receptors in the stomach and vestibular stimulation of the ear, which is one of the primary causes of motion sickness. The side effects of antihistamines include drowsiness, constipation, and dry mouth.

ANXIOLYTICS

Drugs used to treat anxiety are called *anxiolytics* or *antianxiety agents*. The most common class of anxiolytics is the benzodiazepines. These drugs are generally given orally. The benzodiazepines include alprazolam (Xanax), diazepam (Valium), lorazepam (Ativan), and midazolam (Versed). Benzodiazepines are also used as anticonvulsants and muscle relaxers and for symptoms of alcohol (ETOH) withdrawal.

Valium or Versed is often used as a preoperative sedative (given intravenously, intramuscularly, or orally), for induction of anesthesia, or for conscious sedation during interventional procedures. When these two drugs are given intravenously, they may cause respiratory depression, especially when they are used in conjunction with a narcotic. Closely monitor the patient's vital signs, respirations, oxygen saturation level, and level of consciousness.

ANTAGONISTS

The effects of diazepam and midazolam may be reversed using a drug called an *antagonist*. An antagonist inhibits the action of its associated drug. Until recently there were no benzodiazepine antagonists. Now flumazenil (Mazicon or Romazicon), which is used intravenously, stops the effects of benzodiazepines (primarily respiratory depression). Another drug, naloxone (Narcan), is a narcotic antagonist used to reverse respiratory depression caused by narcotic overdose.

ANTICOAGULANTS

Anticoagulants reduce the clotting time of or "thin" the blood. Although they inhibit the clotting mechanisms of the blood, they do not break down or dissolve clots once they have formed (see p. 177).

The two most common anticoagulants are heparin and warfarin (Coumadin). Heparin is usually administered while a patient is hospitalized. It is given intravenously by an infusion pump to ensure correct dosage. Heparin is measured in units, not milligrams. Warfarin may be given orally, and the patient does not have to be hospitalized to receive it. Anticoagulant therapy must be monitored by blood tests that measure factors such as prothrombin time (PT) and activated partial thromboplastin time (APTT).

PT is measured by a blood test and is used to monitor the blood's clotting time. The normal PT is 12 seconds. The therapeutic PT range while a patient is receiving warfarin therapy is from 14 to 18 seconds or as determined by the laboratory. Patients receiving warfarin therapy should have blood tests measuring their PTs performed every day if they are inpatients or every 1 to 4 weeks if they are outpatients to monitor their coagulation times.

APTT, another measure of clotting time, has a normal range of 30 to 45 seconds. The therapeutic APTT range while a patient is receiving heparin therapy is $1\frac{1}{2}$ to $2\frac{1}{2}$ times the control (which is approximately 60 to 135 seconds).

Aspirin may be used to prevent arterial thromboembolisms. Its action is different from heparin or warfarin in that it inhibits platelet aggregation. Because of this, it is classified as an antiplatelet drug. Aspirin may also be used with warfarin to prevent thromboembolisms caused by atrial fibrillation.

ALERT! Patients on any of the anticoagulant drugs mentioned must be monitored closely for signs of bleeding gums, melena (dark, tarry stool), hematuria (blood in urine), bleeding from injection sites or wounds, and bruising.

ANTAGONISTS

Protamine sulfate is an antagonist that neutralizes the effects of heparin. Vitamin K (AquaMEPHYTON) reverses the effects of warfarin, although this may take several hours.

THROMBOLYTIC AGENTS

Thrombolysis, or dissolution of a clot in a vessel, may be accomplished with streptokinase or urokinase. Infusing either of these drugs into the body dissolves the clot's fibrin. These drugs can be used to dissolve fresh clots in blood vessels and, if successful, prevent the need for operations. These agents are often used when performing interventional procedures.

LOCAL ANESTHETICS

Local anesthetics block nerve conduction to anesthetize an area of the body without causing patients to lose consciousness as they do with general anesthetics. Local anesthetics may be administered topically or by injection. Lidocaine is a local anesthetic often used in the radiology department and is also used as an antiarrhythmic medication, particularly for premature ventricular contractions (PVCs). Therefore when administering lidocaine, you must use the appropriate type and strength requested for local anesthesia. Lidocaine also is available in combination with epinephrine. Epinephrine causes vasoconstriction of nearby blood vessels, thus reducing bleeding and localizing the anesthetic effect to an immediate area. Lidocaine is available in several strengths and may be referred to by several names (including lidocaine and xylocaine), so be familiar with which type your department uses.

ANTICHOLINERGICS

Atropine sulfate and glycopyrrolate are the anticholinergic drugs most commonly encountered in radiology departments. Anticholinergic drugs affect the parasympathetic nervous system by blocking the effects of acetylcholine on smooth muscle and glands. In addition, because anticholinergic drugs affect the parasympathetic nervous system, they block the vagal effect on the sinoatrial node of the heart, enhancing electrical conduction through the atrioventricular node and therefore increasing the heart rate. Anticholinergics decrease exocrine gland secretions in the respiratory tract, gastric and salivary glands, and sweat glands, so a patient taking anticholinergic drugs may sweat less and complain of a dry mouth. These drugs also relax all nonvascular smooth muscles, thereby slowing GI and urinary tract activity and possibly causing constipation and urinary retention. For these reasons, anticholinergic drugs may be administered preoperatively to prevent bradycardia and decrease secretions. In addition, they are used to treat symptomatic bradycardia.

PREPARING MEDICATIONS

Follow these guidelines when preparing medications for administration, regardless of the type of dispenser (vial or ampule) used:
1. Use aseptic technique when preparing and administering the medication.
2. Take universal precautions when administering the medication.
3. Choose the correct syringe size according to the amount of medication needed.
4. Maintain the sterility of the syringe and needle connection.
5. Check the physician's order.
6. Read the medication label 3 times: before and after drawing up the medication and before administering the medication.
7. Check the expiration date before preparing the medication for administration.
8. Check the patient's identification.

9. Keep the medication dispenser (vial or ampule) until the completion of the procedure.
10. Dispose of the needle and syringe in a puncture-proof sharps container after use.

VIALS

Vials are single-dose or multidose glass containers with rubber stoppers. A metal cap protects the stopper until the medication is ready for use. Vials contain liquid or powdered medication. The powder must be reconstituted with a solvent before use. Some vials, shaped like hourglasses, contain both a powder and a solvent, with each in its own container. A rubber stopper separates the two compartments. To mix the powder and the solvent, push the uppermost stopper down to create pressure in the vial and dislodge the stopper in the neck between the two compartments. Then mix the solvent and powder with a gentle rotating motion. Procedure 8-1 describes how to draw up medication from a vial.

AMPULES

An **ampule** contains a single dose of liquid medication and varies in size from 1 ml to 10 ml or more. An ampule is made of glass; its narrow, scored neck is snapped off to open it and allow access to the medication (Procedure 8-2). Dispose of the top of the ampule in the sharps container. Unlike drawing medication from vials, you do not need to inject air into ampules to withdraw the medication. Because of capillary action, the medication will not run out of the ampule when it is inverted. Aspirate the contents by pulling back on the syringe plunger. When you have completed the procedure, properly dispose of the ampule in the sharps container.

SAFETY WITH NEEDLES

Accidental needle sticks that occur while recapping needles are one of the most common dangerous incidents in health care settings. OSHA regulations prohibit recapping needles except when using the one-handed method (see Procedure 8-1). The needleless Interlink Vial Access System by Baxter Health Care avoids the use of traditional needles to withdraw medications (Fig. 8-3). IV piggyback tubing can be connected safely to IV injection ports using the Lever Lock (Fig. 8-4); these self-sealing ports can be used repeatedly with the blunt Interlink Cannula (Fig. 8-5).

Text continued on p. 184.

PROCEDURE 8-1
DRAWING UP MEDICATION FROM A VIAL

1. Wash your hands.
2. Open a sterile syringe package and sterile needle package. Place the needle on the syringe, maintaining the sterility of the connection. Do not remove the protective covering from the needle.
3. Check the label to verify you have the correct medication.

4. Remove the metal or plastic cap from the vial without breaking the outside metal seal, and clean the exposed rubber seal with an alcohol wipe.

5. Remove the needle cap. Pull a portion of air into the syringe that is equal to the amount of medication to be aspirated.

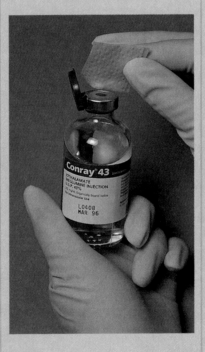

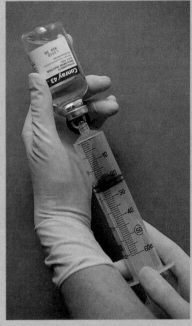

6. Insert the needle into the center of the rubber seal.
7. Invert the vial with your nondominant hand, and inject air into the vial.

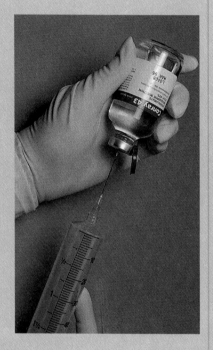

ALERT! To avoid breaking the vial with air pressure, never inject more air into the vial than the total contents of the vial.

8. Grasp the end of the barrel and plunger of the syringe with your dominant thumb and forefinger, and gently pull the contents into the syringe, keeping the tip of the needle below the fluid level.

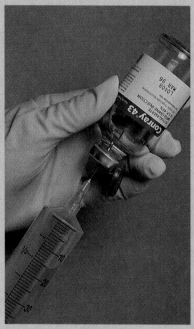

9. When the correct amount of medication is obtained, remove the needle from the vial by pulling back on the syringe barrel.
10. Tap the syringe gently to dislodge air bubbles toward the hub of the syringe, and gently depress the plunger to expel the air without ejecting the medication.
11. If the needle must be recapped, place the cap on the counter, and with your dominant hand holding the syringe, insert the needle into the cap.

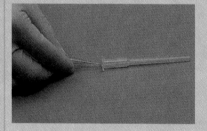

12. Wash your hands.

PROCEDURE 8-2
PREPARING MEDICATION FROM AN AMPULE

1. Wash your hands.
2. Open a sterile syringe package and sterile needle package. Place the needle on the syringe, maintaining the sterility of the connection. Do not remove the protective covering from the needle.
3. Check the label to verify you have the correct medication.
4. Tap the top of the ampule lightly with your finger until fluid leaves the neck of the ampule.
5. If the ampule is not scored, partially file the neck of the ampule to ensure a clean break.

6. Using gauze or a dry alcohol wipe, grasp the top or stem of the ampule with your dominant hand. Grasp the bottom of the ampule with your nondominant hand.

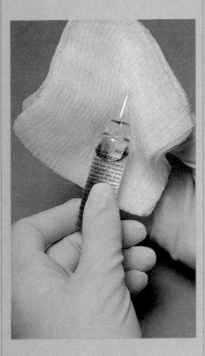

7. With a quick, firm action, snap the neck away from you.
8. Either invert the ampule or set it on a flat surface to withdraw the medication.
9. Keep the needle below the level of the liquid and gently pull back on the plunger of the syringe. Do not force air into the syringe, since this will cause the medication to run out.

10. Tip the ampule as needed to bring all fluid within reach of the needle.

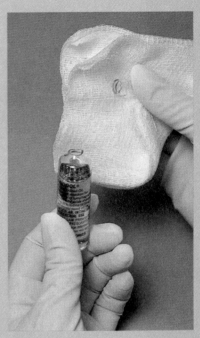

11. To expel excess air from the syringe, remove the syringe from the ampule. Hold the syringe with the needle up and tap it to force air bubbles to the top of the syringe. Expel the air, and reinsert the syringe into the ampule to withdraw the remainder of the medication.
12. Change the needle on the syringe.
13. Dispose of the needle and ampule top in the sharps container.
14. Wash your hands.

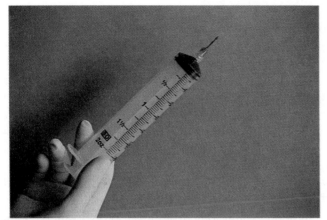

FIG. 8-3 Interlink vial access cannula. (Courtesy Baxter Health Care.)

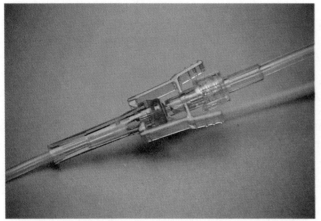

FIG. 8-4 Needleless system interlink lever lock for IV piggyback medication administration. (Courtesy Baxter Health Care.)

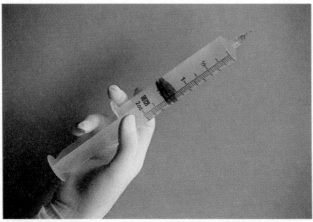

FIG. 8-5 Interlink syringe cannula. (Courtesy Baxter Health Care.)

VENIPUNCTURE

Venipuncture is performed by many radiologic technologists to administer contrast media. In many states, only radiologists and nurses perform venipuncture for contrast administration. Although in some states technologists are allowed to perform venipuncture, some hospital policies still prohibit that this practice be performed by anyone in the radiology department except physicians and registered nurses. It is important for you to know your state's standards as well as the policies of your employer before performing venipuncture.

The American Society of Radiologic Technologists (ASRT) has mandated that venipuncture techniques be included in the curriculum of radiologic technology programs. Some hospitals require new technologists to complete venipuncture courses before they are allowed to perform venipuncture in their specific institution, regardless of prior experience at other institutions. Venipuncture courses should address the way to perform the procedure and review various types of contrast media, contrast reactions, complications of venipuncture, emergency equipment, types of needles used, and basic venous anatomy.

PREPARING FOR VENIPUNCTURE

Venipuncture may cause a great deal of anxiety in patients, especially in those who have had unpleasant experiences with it in the past or whose venous anatomy makes venipuncture difficult. Be calm and confident to help put patients at ease. Be prepared and have all necessary equipment readily available so that you will not have to stop the procedure to look for supplies.

Have the following equipment ready:
- Alcohol prep or povidone-iodine prep (depending on institution policy)
- Tourniquet
- Cotton balls
- Tape
- Gloves
- Needles (Have more than one of each size and type available.)
- Syringe with contrast media
- Adhesive strip or gauze for dressing
- Folded towel

Choose a needle or an over-the-needle catheter based on your familiarity with the needle, the amount of time the needle will remain in place, and the purpose of the injection. Over-the-needle catheters (Angiocath or Jelco) are generally used for IV lines that will remain in place but may be used for injection of contrast media by a power injector (as used in computed tomography). Butterfly needles are often used for bolus contrast injections.

The needle size, or gauge, is determined by the size of the vein and the intended purpose of the needle. Usually 20 to 22 gauge needles are adequate for IV fluids and contrast administration. Larger gauge needles, such as 16 to 18 gauge, are used for surgery and administering blood and blood products. Smaller gauge needles, such as 22 to 25 gauge, are used for children and infants.

VEIN SELECTION

When locating the best vein for venipuncture, keep in mind whether it is for short- or long-term use. The general rule is to start looking for veins distally; that is, begin looking in the area around the patient's hand or forearm. (Fig. 8-6 shows the veins commonly used for venipuncture.) If the sole purpose of the venipuncture is to inject contrast material (short-term use), the antecubital space usually has the largest veins. If the needle or catheter will remain in place for any length of time, avoid this area, since it is difficult to maintain patency when the patient's arm is bent.

Choose the best vein by observation and palpation. Place a tourniquet 7 to 10 cm (3 to 4 inches) above the intended site to engorge and dilate the veins.

The vein should feel soft and relatively spongy, not hard. Visually follow the course of the vein to make sure it is not full of turns and bends (tortuous). Locate hard-to-find veins by applying a warm compress, allowing the patients' arms to dangle, or having patients open and close their fists.

Avoid the following types of veins:
1. Veins that are tortuous or hard to see or palpate
2. Repeatedly used veins
3. Veins in areas where the skin is not in good condition (rashes, bruises, scarring, infected)
4. Veins that lay on an artery (for example, the brachial artery medial to the antecubital space)
5. Thin, superficial veins
6. Areas near bifurcating (branching) veins
7. Veins in extremities compromised by surgery (such as distal amputation, mastectomy, or dialysis shunt)
8. Veins in extremities compromised by a cerebral vascular accident
9. Areas of the wrist or antecubital fossa where flexion may cause catheter occlusion or dislodging of the needle from the vein

After selecting the appropriate vein, follow the steps listed in Procedure 8-3 to perform the venipuncture.

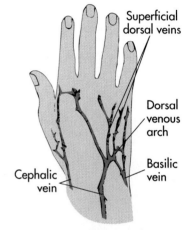

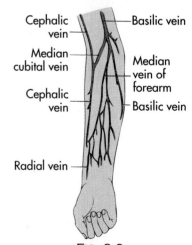

FIG. 8-6
Veins easily accessible for venipuncture.

PROCEDURE 8-3
VENIPUNCTURE

1. Wash your hands.
2. Introduce yourself to the patient, and check the patient's identification band.
3. Address the patient by name, and explain the procedure and the reason it is being done.
4. Ask the patient to remain still during the procedure.
5. Determine the best site for the venipuncture.
6. Cleanse the skin with alcohol or povidone-iodine in a circular motion, starting in the middle and working out to a radius of about 5 cm (2 inches).

8. Verify you have the proper medication.
9. Put on gloves.
10. Anchor the vein with your nondominant hand or thumb to prevent movement and make the skin taut. This allows easier needle insertion.
11. With the bevel of the needle facing up, puncture the skin at a 20 to 45° angle with a quick motion, and insert the needle farther until you feel it pop through the vein. Blood should enter the flash chamber or tubing, indicating that you have entered the vein.

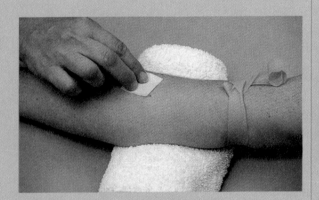

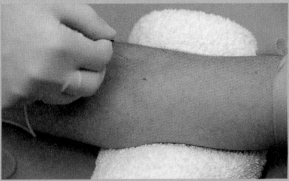

7. Apply a tourniquet 7 to 10 cm (3 to 4 inches) above the site.

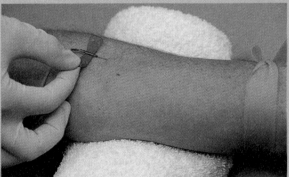

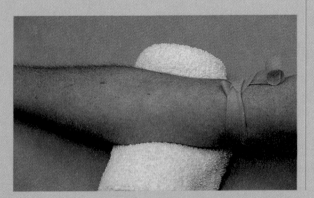

12. Decrease the angle of the needle, and insert the needle or catheter ¼ to ½ inch farther into the vein. If you are using an over-the-needle catheter, slowly withdraw the stylet as you insert the catheter. Do not touch the needle or catheter as you insert the needle through the skin; this may allow bacteria to enter the skin with the needle.

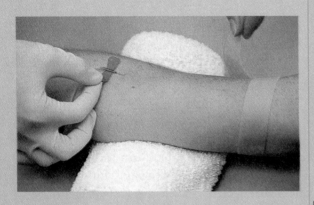

13. Release the tourniquet and attach IV tubing, or if injecting contrast material with a butterfly and syringe, proceed with the injection. Tape the butterfly in place while injecting to prevent the needle from dislodging.

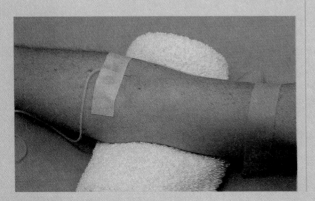

14. *Note:* In some institutions, technologists are taught to perform a venipuncture as a method for starting an IV drip. In this case, follow your institution's policies for site dressings. Always label the site with the size of needle, the date, and your initials.

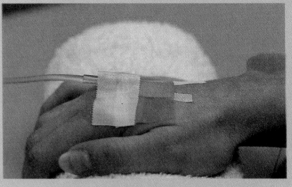

ALERT! If the venipuncture is unsuccessful, withdraw the needle or catheter, and immediately apply light pressure to the insertion site with a cotton ball or gauze. When reattempting a venipuncture, *always* use a new needle.

PRINCIPLES FOR VENIPUNCTURE

Do not reuse a catheter or needle.

Always wear gloves and take universal precautions during a venipuncture or discontinuation of an IV line.

Dispose of needles and catheters in proper containers.

Although catheters and needleless systems are not sharp, they are considered contaminated and universal precautions must be taken to dispose of them.

Notify nursing personnel if the dressing on an IV becomes loose or saturated. The dressing over an IV site should remain sterile, dry, and intact.

If a needle or catheter becomes dislodged, do not attempt to push it back into the vein. Notify nursing personnel or discontinue the IV line.

INFILTRATION

A needle or catheter can become dislodged, or a needle can puncture a wall of a vein. Either situation causes an **infiltration** (also called *extravasation*) of fluid into surrounding tissues. Fluid has infiltrated the tissues if patients have the following symptoms:

1. Swelling or redness at the site
2. Cool skin at the site
3. A pressure sensation or burning at the site
4. No blood return

If infiltration occurs, withdraw the needle or catheter and dispose of it properly. Apply a warm compress to the site. Document the infiltration according to your institution's standards. The box summarizes the principles for venipuncture.

CONTRAST MEDIA

Contrast agents are often used to image different organs. Because many body parts show little contrast on nonenhanced radiographs and images, the use of contrast agents improves the radiographic visualization. Contrast media are used in radiographic procedures, fluoroscopic procedures, computed tomographic procedures, cardiovascular-interventional procedures, and magnetic resonance procedures. Radiographers encounter a variety of contrast agents daily (Fig. 8-7). Contrast agents may be classified as either **positive contrast media** or **negative contrast media**.

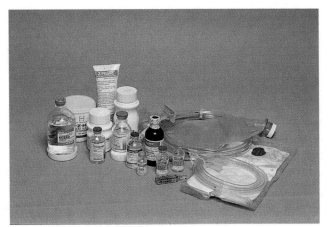

FIG. 8-7 Common contrast agents used in radiology.

NEGATIVE CONTRAST MEDIA

Negative contrast materials may be used for procedures such as double-contrast GI studies and arthrograms. These agents have very low atomic numbers and are easily penetrated by x-rays. This causes an increase in the photographic density of the finished radiographic image, so the anatomic areas filled by negative contrast agents appear black.

The most common negative contrast agent used is air. However, carbon dioxide, oxygen, and nitrous oxide may also be used. When introduced into a body part, negative contrast agents are almost always used in combination with positive contrast agents (which cause anatomic areas to appear lighter) to improve visualization of specific structures.

Air is normally found within body parts such as the lungs and bowel, so the radiologist can depend on normal air patterns to assist in the diagnosis of abnormal conditions. In such cases, additional negative contrast agents are not needed. For example, air within the pleural cavity is not normal and indicates the presence of a pneumothorax. In addition, bowel obstructions are clearly visible on plain abdominal radiographs because of alterations in the normal bowel gas patterns.

POSITIVE CONTRAST MEDIA

Positive contrast media have high atomic numbers and prevent x-rays from reaching film. This causes a decrease in the photographic density of the finished radiographic image, so the image appears light. In most departments, you will encounter a variety of positive contrast agents daily. Different positive contrast agents are administered orally, intravenously, intraarterially, and intrathecally. These agents include barium sulfate products, iodinated products, and gadolinium products.

BARIUM SULFATE

Barium sulfate ($BaSO_4$) in a water suspension is the most common positive contrast agent used to image the GI system. Barium, a heavy metal with an atomic number of 56, is not water soluble, so barium sulfate is suspended when mixed with water. When left for a period of time, the barium sulfate will sink to the bottom of the container.

Administer barium sulfate orally for esophagus, stomach, and small bowel studies. When performing large bowel studies, administer barium sulfate via an enema. Barium sulfate contrast agents are available in a variety of concentrations from several pharmaceutical companies. Each variety has a specific use for enhancing the GI system and may be used in combination with a negative contrast agent. Barium sulfate administered by enemas should be mixed with cold tap water to reduce colonic spasms and cramping.

Because barium sulfate is not water soluble, it cannot be naturally absorbed by the body. It should never be injected into the bloodstream or subarachnoid space and should never be used in a location where it can leak into the peritoneal cavity. Therefore if there is any possibility there is a bowel perforation, a water-soluble, iodinated contrast agent should be used.

Give patients instructions on preparing for the procedure. (Preparation varies with specific procedures.) In addition, provide follow-up care before they leave the department. Patients should be informed that barium sulfate contrast agents may cause constipation. Therefore they should be instructed to drink plenty of fluids after the procedure and to use mild laxatives if necessary. A bowel obstruction can result if the barium sulfate is not eliminated from the body and hardens within the bowel.

IODINATED CONTRAST PRODUCTS

Iodinated contrast agents are the most commonly used contrast agents in radiology departments. These contrast agents are used in radiographic studies of the urinary system, a multitude of fluoroscopic procedures, all cardiovascular-interventional studies, and many computed tomographic studies. Iodine has a fairly high atomic number, so it is an excellent positive contrast agent. Iodinated contrast agents may be administered orally, intravenously, intraarterially, or intrathecally, depending on the procedure. They may be water soluble or oil based and ionic or nonionic.

OIL-BASED CONTRAST AGENTS **Oil-based contrast agents** may be used in studies of the female reproductive system via hysterosalpingography and the lymphatic system via lymphography. The oil base is not water soluble and should *never* be injected into the bloodstream, which would create an embolism—a fatal complication. Oil-based contrast agents have limited use in modern imaging departments.

WATER-SOLUBLE CONTRAST AGENTS **Water-soluble contrast agents** are the most commonly employed positive contrast agents in most radiology departments. These drugs may be administered orally, intravascularly, rectally, or by injection into body cavities for radiographic visualization. As mentioned previously, water-soluble contrast materials should be used to visualize a bowel when there is a possibility it is perforated.

Water-soluble contrast agents are the only type of contrast materials that can be injected into the bloodstream. When iodinated contrast agents are injected into the bloodstream or subarachnoid space, they are excreted through the kidneys within 24 hr, with peak urine concentrations occurring within the first hour.

Water-soluble contrast agents are classified as ionic or nonionic and are available in various iodine concentrations. As the iodine concentration increases, so does the radioopacity of the visualized structure. However, greater iodine concentrations also result in a higher viscosity and risk of toxicity. Vascular injection of water-soluble contrast agents frequently causes a sensation of warmth. Patients may also experience nausea, vomiting, urticarial patches (hives), and edema in the respiratory mucous membrane. Severe reactions, including anaphylactoid, cardiovascular, and central nervous system reactions, may also occur.

Take the proper precautions before injecting contrast materials. Most contrast reactions occur within the first 5 minutes of injection. All patients, however, should be monitored for 1 hr after injection because delayed reactions can occur.

Obtain a thorough medical history from patients before administering contrast agents. The history must include the following information:

• Previous reactions to contrast material
• Sensitivity to iodine
• A history of bronchial asthma or hay fever
• Known food or medication allergies

Also obtain preprocedure vital signs (blood pressure, respirations, and pulse) to serve as baseline measurements before the injection. The patient's history and vital signs must be clearly and correctly documented.

Ionic contrast agents **Ionic contrast agents** consist of a benzene ring that combines organic iodine with sodium salts or methylglucamine (meglumine) salts. When injected into the bloodstream, the benzene ring structure partially disassociates into ionic particles known as *anions* (−) and *cations* (+), which is why it is an ionic agent. The resulting electrolyte imbalance causes fluid to be drawn into the bloodstream from the surrounding tissues, which is believed by some researchers to increase the risk of adverse reactions to ionic agents. For this reason, nonionic contrast agents were developed. They became commercially available in the 1980s.

Nonionic contrast agents **Nonionic contrast agents** also contain iodine. Their molecular structure, however, does not disassociate when it is injected into the bloodstream. Because nonionic contrast materials cause fewer adverse reactions than ionic contrast materials, they are frequently used for high-risk patients and procedures. Nonionic contrast agents include iohexol, iopamidol, and ioversol products. They can be used intravenously for urographic, computed tomographic, and fluoroscopic studies; intrathecally for myelographic and computed tomographic studies of the spine; and intraarterially for angiographic studies.

GADOLINIUM CONTRAST AGENTS

Gadolinium contrast agents are only used for magnetic resonance examinations. They enhance visualization of certain pathologic conditions that otherwise may not be clearly seen. The physician who interprets the examination determines whether to use gadolinium.

SUMMARY

As a health care professional, you are responsible for administering medication safely and effectively. You must adhere to state laws and institutional policies and procedures. The preparation and administration of medication requires accuracy. If a drug is administered incorrectly, it can harm the patient; therefore always verify the *five rights* when administering a drug. These are the right medication, right dose, right patient, right route, and right time. Be sure to obtain a thorough medical history, including allergy information, before administering medications, and be prepared to respond to adverse reactions should they occur. Patients' well-being depends on your knowledge and practice of the basic principles of medication administration.

STUDY QUESTIONS

1. What are the technologist's responsibilities when administering any medication?
2. What part do the kidneys play in the metabolism of drugs?
3. Does the route of administration alter the dosage of a drug? If so, in what way?
4. What effects do corticosteroids and epinephrine have on patients, experiencing contrast reactions?
5. Why is aspirin sometimes called a "blood thinner"?
6. What determines the size and type of needle used for a venipuncture?
7. What steps may be taken to adequately locate an acceptable vein for a venipuncture?
8. What should be done if a contrast agent infiltrates the tissues?
9. What is the most commonly used negative contrast agent? In what way does it appear on a radiograph?
10. Name two uses for barium sulfate.
11. What type or types of contrast media may be used when performing intravenous urography studies?
12. What are the advantages of using nonionic contrast agents when performing studies that require vascular injections?

Nine

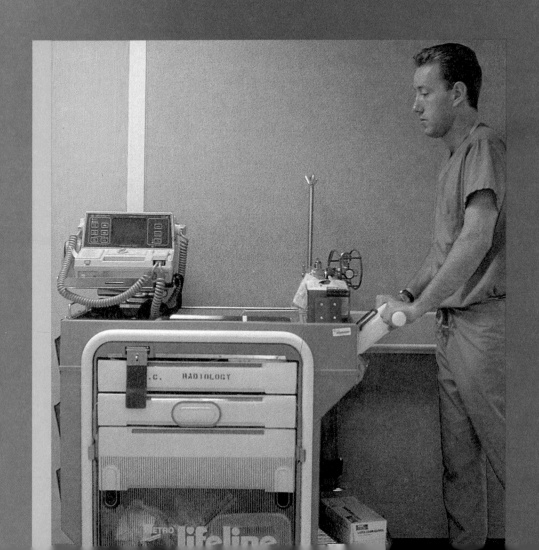

Patient Care in Critical Situations

Key Terms

Contents

Objectives

AFTER COMPLETING THIS CHAPTER, THE STUDENT WILL BE ABLE TO:

1. Explain the way to prioritize patient care according to immediate needs.
2. Describe the typical contents of an emergency crash cart.
3. Demonstrate the ability to assist a code team during a cardiac or respiratory arrest.
4. Describe four factors that may alter a patient's respiratory status.
5. Demonstrate the way to open a patient's airway.
6. Identify the universal sign for choking.
7. Explain the reason an oxygen mask is used in certain situations instead of a nasal cannula.
8. Demonstrate the ability to care for a patient having a seizure.
9. Describe the signs and symptoms of a patient with an altered level of consciousness.
10. List five possible causes of fainting.
11. Describe the signs and symptoms of shock.
12. Demonstrate the ability to care for a patient having a diabetic emergency.
13. Explain how insulin affects blood glucose levels.

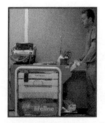

IMAGING TECHNOLOGISTS MAY ENCOUNTER A variety of unexpected changes in patient status (especially in emergency rooms) resulting from certain types of procedures (such as fluoroscopic and cardiovascular-interventional radiologic), illness, or injury. Unexpected changes in patient status range from developing mild conditions, such as urticaria (hives) after the injection of a contrast agent, to life-threatening conditions, such as having a cardiac arrest. Even events that begin as mild, nonemergency situations can escalate into life-threatening crises in debilitated patients. To prevent further injury or deterioration of a patient's condition, you must be able to recognize changes in the patient's medical status and respond immediately and appropriately. You need to be calm and confident and handle each situation professionally, efficiently, and appropriately.

Being prepared begins with knowing where emergency equipment and supplies are kept. Your responses to acute and life-threatening situations *do* affect patients' outcomes. It is everyone's responsibility to assist in preserving a patient's life. When emergencies arise, you must obtain appropriate medical assistance as quickly as possible. In some situations, you may be required to initiate a treatment such as cardiopulmonary resuscitation (CPR). In other situations, you can only protect the patient from further harm, such as assisting a patient who has fainted or is having a seizure.

EMERGENCY CHANGES IN PATIENT STATUS

Patient status refers to a patient's physiologic status in key categories including consciousness, oxygenation, and circulation. Changes in any of these categories of status often require life-saving interventions to restore physiologic equilibrium. Such interventions may include starting CPR, assisting with administering emergency medications, and restraining confused or violent patients. As discussed previously, remembering the most basic human needs (in Maslow's hierarchy) helps you prioritize your actions when caring for patients. Any threat to a patient's airway, breathing, or circulation is considered a top priority and requires immediate attention.

In patients with obstructed airways or difficulty breathing, the oxygen concentration in the bloodstream declines, resulting in insufficient oxygenation of the body tissues and organs. An organ deprived of oxygen may be irreversibly damaged in a matter of minutes. Respiratory arrest progresses to loss of consciousness and cardiac arrest unless the obstruction is removed and artificial respirations are administered. Respiratory and cardiac arrests are critical, life-threatening emergencies you must be prepared to handle at any time. Technologists must be certified in basic life support CPR. Most medical facilities have a specified group of health care professionals (physicians, nurses, respiratory therapists, and pharmacists) trained to respond to cardiac and respiratory arrests. This group is often referred to as the *code team*.

Some patients are at a higher risk for having a cardiac or respiratory arrest, such as patients with cardiopulmonary illnesses or severe electrolyte disturbances. Before beginning invasive procedures or injecting patients with contrast agents, obtain a thorough medical history, including information about any existing cardiac arrhythmias, and assess baseline vital signs. An irregular cardiac rhythm in a patient with a cardiovascular disease such as coronary artery disease or who has had a myocardial infarction or open-heart surgery can quickly progress to a cardiac arrest.

If a patient has a cardiac or respiratory arrest in the imaging department, you have the responsibility to assist the code team in any way possible. Provide as much information as possible to the team about the events leading up to the arrest. After making sure that all emergency equipment has been brought to the team (suction equip-

EQUIPMENT AND SUPPLIES ON A CODE CART

MEDICATIONS

Drugs, needles, and syringes

AIRWAY EQUIPMENT

Laryngoscopes, endotracheal tubes, ambu bag, oxygen tubing, suction catheters, and portable suction machine

CIRCULATION EQUIPMENT

IV solutions and tubing, IV cannulas, cut-down tray, blood gas kits, and blood collection tubes

MISCELLANEOUS

Backboard, stethoscope, blood pressure cuff, flashlight, extension cord, needle box

PROTECTIVE EQUIPMENT

Sterile and nonsterile gloves, protective eyewear, masks, gowns

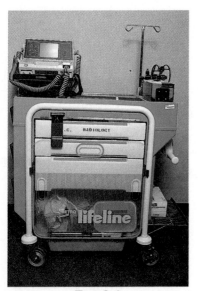

FIG. 9-1
Emergency cart with defibrillator.

ment, a defibrillator, a code cart, and oxygen), you can assist with documentation. Record the time of arrest, time and name of medications given, time and frequency of defibrillations, vital signs, and cardiac rhythm. Other helpful tasks include calling the patient's floor, the laboratory, or clergy; stamping paperwork with the patient's addressograph plate; and taking specimens to the laboratory.

EMERGENCY EQUIPMENT

You must know the location of all emergency equipment in your imaging department, including the crash cart, oxygen, emergency medications, and suction equipment.

In-service education classes should be held regularly to reorient technologists and others about the location and contents of emergency carts. Most carts contain basic supplies, drugs, and documentation forms used in code situations and are organized fairly consistently and logically (box). The cart has wheels for easy transportation and may have an attached defibrillator (Fig. 9-1).

AIRWAY AND BREATHING

Breathing is both a voluntary and an involuntary bodily function. It is easy and automatic unless physical stressors interfere, such as disease processes (masses, infectious processes, edema, and chronic obstructive pulmonary disease [COPD]), irritants (such as gases and microorganisms), physical size (obesity), trauma, physical deformities, or physical exercise. Respirations may also be altered by drugs such as narcotics and benzodiazepines that cause respiratory depression. Breathing can also be impeded by choking caused by a foreign body in the airway.

Maintaining a clear airway is one of your highest priorities and can be as simple as repositioning patients to help them breathe more comfortably. Patients who are obese or pregnant often cannot lie on their backs because their weight presses on their diaphragms and makes breathing difficult. They should be positioned upright or on their right sides.

Any patient who seems short of breath or whose color is cyanotic (bluish around the lips, ears, and nailbeds) should be checked immediately for respiratory distress. Irregular breathing patterns, high-pitched inspiratory noises, and wheezing are all signs of respiratory distress. Ask patients with suspected airway obstructions to speak to you. Individuals with total airway obstructions are completely unable to speak. If a patient can speak and cough forcefully, no immediate intervention is necessary; encourage the person to keep coughing to clear the airway. If a patient is unable to speak or cannot cough forcefully enough to dislodge an obstruction, immediately intervene with the Heimlich maneuver (described on p. 203). Respiratory distress is often increased by anxiety, so try to keep the patient calm.

Unconscious patients' tongues or dentures may obstruct their airways. In addition, patients with diminished or absent gag and cough reflexes are more likely to aspirate if they vomit or drink contrast agents. Vomitus in the mouth or on the face may be a sign of foreign body airway obstruction that needs immediate attention.

RESPIRATORY ARREST

If a patient is not breathing—a condition called **respiratory arrest**—activate the emergency system. See Procedure 9-1 for the way to open an airway and perform rescue breathing.

OXYGEN THERAPY

You may be required to change a patient's oxygen tank if it is almost empty or provide a patient with oxygen therapy at a physician's request. You should know where oxygen and oxygen delivery supplies are kept (Figs. 9-2 and 9-3). Also familiarize yourself with the way to check and change the flow meter/regulator on an oxygen tank. In

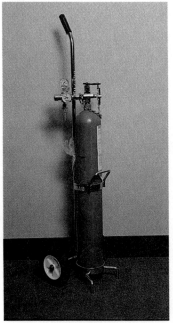

FIG. 9-2
Oxygen tank.

PROCEDURE 9-1
RESCUE BREATHING

1. Place one hand on the patient's forehead.
2. Use your other hand to lift the patient's chin and tip the head back to open the airway. If there is a possibility the patient has a head or neck trauma, use the jaw-thrust maneuver instead.

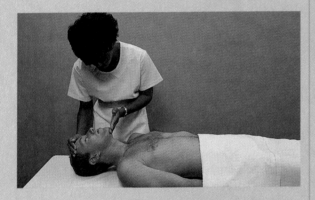

3. Look, listen, and feel for breathing for 3 to 5 seconds.

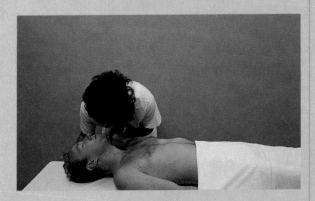

4. If the patient is still not breathing, start rescue breathing. Cover the patient's mouth with your mouth and pinch the nose shut, or use a mask to provide ventilations.

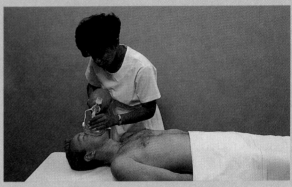

5. Give the patient a full, slow breath every 5 seconds (every 3 seconds for children and infants). Check to see that the chest rises with each breath to ensure adequate ventilation.
6. If you are unsuccessful in ventilating the patient's lungs, readjust the head to open the airway and try to ventilate again.
7. If you are still unsuccessful, perform the Heimlich maneuver or a maneuver for clearing a foreign body from an obstructed airway as described in Procedures 9-2 and 9-3.
8. Every minute or so, monitor the patient's pulse to verify there is circulation.
9. Continue until help comes or the patient recovers.

   Note: In patients with tracheostomies, you must ventilate the lungs through the stoma instead of the mouth. You may also ventilate the lungs through the nose for patients in whom mouth-to-mouth ventilations are contraindicated, such as patients with facial injuries or vomitus in or around the mouth.

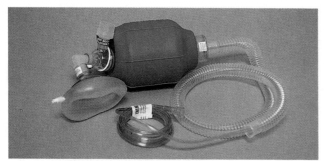

FIG. 9-3 Ambu bag with oxygen tubing.

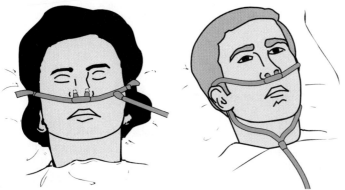

FIG. 9-4 Nasal cannula. (Modified from Potter PA, Perry AG, *Fundamentals of nursing: concepts, process, and practice*, ed 3, St Louis, 1994, Mosby.)

many hospitals the respiratory therapy department is responsible for initiating and maintaining oxygen therapy. The respiratory therapist who is responsible for the patient can show you the way to change tanks and properly store oxygen equipment and supplies.

Oxygen may be administered by a nasal cannula or mask. Nasal cannulas (Fig. 9-4) are for low oxygen concentrations (1 to 6 L O_2/min). A cannula is less constricting than a face mask, although it dries out the nasal mucous membranes and causes nasal congestion.

The simple face mask (Fig. 9-5) consists of a plastic mask with air vents on the side to allow for a mixture of room air with oxygen and the release of expired air. This type of mask can deliver 4 to 6 L O_2/min.

A nonrebreather mask is used for high-concentration oxygen administration and prevents expired air from mixing with administered oxygen. Expired air is vented out the mask through exhalation

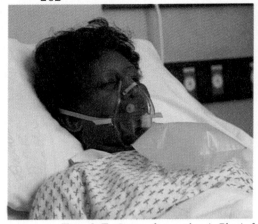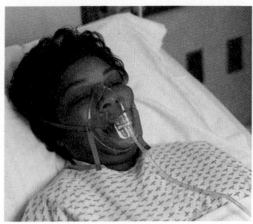

FIG. 9-5 Oxygen face masks. **A,** Plastic face mask with reservoir bag. **B,** Simple face mask. (From Potter PA, Perry AG, *Fundamentals of nursing: concepts, process, and practice,* ed 3, St Louis, 1994, Mosby.)

ports. This mask is uncomfortable and designed for short-term use only.

Venturi masks are often used for patients with COPD who cannot tolerate high oxygen concentrations. (Higher oxygen concentrations diminish the hypoxic respiratory drive to breathe.) Oxygen is forced through a small opening, which increases its velocity and pulls air into the mask to mix with the oxygen.

Some patients must have a mechanical ventilator to maintain their breathing. In most cases, patients being transported to imaging departments on ventilators have respiratory therapists accompanying them to monitor their conditions and ventilators. In units where you perform portable radiography, however, a respiratory therapist may not always be with the patient. Notify a nurse or respiratory therapist (if one is available) if any alarms sound, especially while you are positioning a patient. Tubing can become disconnected, or the physical movement may cause the patient respiratory distress.

CHOKING

Technologists must be able to recognize and respond quickly to a choking patient. As described earlier, a patient who is choking cannot speak. The universal sign for choking is clutching the neck between the thumb and fingers. The **Heimlich maneuver** is used to clear a foreign body obstructing the airway. Follow the steps in Procedure 9-2.

HEIMLICH MANEUVER

SITTING OR STANDING PATIENT

1. Stand behind the patient and put your arms around the patient's body just above the waist.
2. Place the thumb side of one fist against the abdomen midway between the umbilicus and the xiphoid process. Grasp the fist with your other hand.
3. Pull your fists into the abdomen with quick inward and upward thrusts.

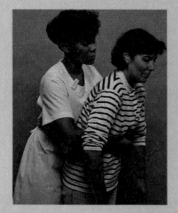

4. Repeat the thrusts up to 5 times or until the patient expels the object or faints. If the patient begins to cough forcefully, stop the maneuver but observe the patient carefully.
5. If patients faint, help them to the floor to avoid injury. Place patients on their backs.

SUPINE (UNCONSCIOUS) PATIENT

1. To perform a finger sweep, open the patient's mouth, grasp the tongue and mandible with your thumb and index finger, and lift up.

Sweep the index finger of your other hand along the cheek to the posterior pharynx to dislodge any foreign bodies.
2. Attempt to ventilate the patient's lungs with the rescue breathing technique.
3. If the ventilation does not successfully enter the patient's lungs, kneel and straddle the patient's thighs.
4. Place the heel of one hand on top of the other against the midabdomen (between the xiphoid process and umbilicus).
5. Give five upward abdominal thrusts, and then check the mouth for the foreign body.
6. Move to the patient's head and attempt to ventilate the lungs again. If this is unsuccessful, continue the sequence of thrusts, sweep, and ventilation until the object is expelled or you have completed four cycles; call for help.
7. If patients begin to vomit, move them onto their sides to prevent aspiration.

OBESE OR PREGNANT PATIENTS (SITTING OR STANDING)

Obese or pregnant patients should receive *chest thrusts* instead of abdominal thrusts.
1. Stand behind the patient, and put your arms around the patient's body just beneath the axilla.
2. Place the thumb side of one fist against the middle portion of the sternum, avoiding the xiphoid process. Grasp the fist with the other hand.
3. Pull your fists into the chest with quick backward thrusts.
4. Repeat this maneuver up to 5 times.

5. If patients faint, help them to the floor to avoid injury. Place patients on their backs, and kneel close to their sides.
6. Place the heel of both hands in the middle of the sternum, and press inward 5 times.
7. Move to the patient's head and attempt to ventilate the lungs. If this is unsuccessful, continue the sequence of thrusts, sweep, and ventilation until the object is expelled or you have completed four cycles; call for help.
8. If patients begin to vomit, move them onto their sides to prevent aspiration.

INFANTS

1. Attempt to ventilate the infant's lungs by covering the mouth and nose with your mouth. If the ventilation attempt is unsuccessful, readjust the head position, and try to ventilate the lungs again.
2. If the second ventilation attempt is unsuccessful, place the infant prone with the head lower than the trunk. You may rest the infant's body along your forearm.
3. Deliver five back blows between the infant's scapulae with the heel of one hand.
4. Support the infant's head, and turn the infant supine. Place two fingers over the lower third of the sternum, and give five downward thrusts.
5. Attempt to ventilate the infant's lungs again. If the ventilation attempt is unsuccessful, continue the sequence of back blows, thrusts, and ventilation until the object is expelled or until you have completed four cycles; call for help.

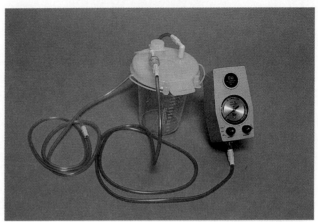

FIG. 9-6 Wall suction apparatus.

SUCTIONING

Signs and symptoms of airway obstructions that may require suctioning include gurgling sounds when inspiring or expiring, drooling, obvious gastric secretions in the mouth, and coughing without clearing secretions. Although having patients try to cough forcefully to clear their airways is preferable, patients with diminished or absent gag and cough reflexes and debilitated or unconscious patients may be unable to clear their airways adequately. In such cases, oropharyngeal or nasopharyngeal suctioning may be performed by someone trained in suctioning procedures. Because respiratory therapists, nurses, and physicians perform this procedure in most institutions, the procedure is not described in detail here.

The equipment for suctioning patients' airways includes in-wall (Fig. 9-6) and portable suction machines, adapters and tubing, suction catheters (10 to 18 F for adults, 5 to 8 F for children), a basin, sterile water or normal saline, a towel, and possibly an oral airway. Keep clean collection devices and tubing with the equipment. Clean, nonsterile gloves and a face shield or goggles should be worn when suctioning to protect against exposure to body fluids.

CARDIOPULMONARY RESUSCITATION

Death from **cardiac arrest,** a condition in which the heart stops beating, can be prevented by immediate **cardiopulmonary resuscitation (CPR).** The signs and symptoms of cardiac arrest are listed in the box.

SIGNS AND SYMPTOMS OF CARDIAC ARREST

- Clutching at chest
- Viselike pain in chest possibly radiating to jaw, neck, or arm
- Sweating, pallor, shortness of breath
- Irregular heartbeat
- Feeling of "indigestion" that does not diminish after using antacids

Because early heart defibrillation in adults has been proved to save lives, the American Heart Association recommends activating the emergency medical system (EMS) as soon as you determine a patient is unresponsive. Immediately follow your institution's protocol for reporting cardiac arrests. If no protocol exists or you are outside the institution, call 9-1-1.

A **defibrillator** is a machine that delivers an electrical shock to a patient to stimulate the heart into a normal electrical rhythm. Two paddles are positioned on the patient's chest—one at the fifth intercostal space on the left midclavicular line and one at the third intercostal space to the right of the sternum. Conducting gel or saline pads are used between the paddles and skin to prevent skin burns and ensure conductance. Members of the code team and others present during the defibrillation must avoid touching the patient or anything in contact with the patient during the procedure. When the equipment is charged and the code team is ready, the person performing the defibrillation announces: "Clear!" to warn everyone to stand clear of the patient and bed or cart.

Procedure 9-3 is an abbreviated description of the procedure for performing adult CPR. Do not try to perform CPR without proper training by and certification from a qualified instructor.

The brain cannot survive without oxygen for more than 4 to 6 minutes; therefore you must initiate CPR immediately after determining that a person's respiratory and cardiac functions have ceased.

ALTERED LEVEL OF CONSCIOUSNESS

A person's consciousness exists on a continuum that ranges from complete awareness and alertness to total unresponsiveness. As a patient's level of consciousness decreases, the patient may seem irritable and uncooperative. If a patient who previously appeared alert and acted appropriately begins to give inappropriate responses

1. Place one hand on the patient's forehead.
2. Use your other hand to lift the patient's chin and tip the head back to open the airway. If there is a possibility the patient has a head or neck trauma, use the jaw thrust maneuver instead.

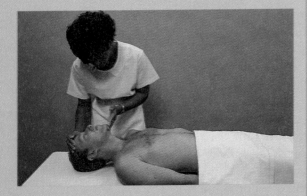

3. Look, listen, and feel for breathing for 3 to 5 seconds.
4. Ventilate the patient's lungs with two full breaths, watching to make sure the chest rises.
5. Check the carotid pulse for 5 to 10 seconds. If there is no pulse, begin chest compressions.

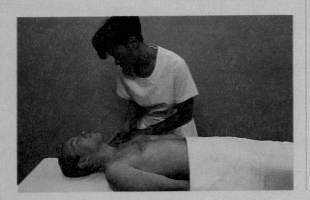

6. Use the following method to correctly position the hands during chest compressions (to avoid breaking the ribs and xiphoid process, which can cause internal injuries). Find the last rib and follow it to the xiphoid process. Place the heel of one hand one or two finger widths above the xiphoid process. Place the heel of your other hand on top of the first.
7. Keep your elbows straight and begin compressing the chest 3.5 to 5 cm (1½ to 2 inches) with a ratio of 15 compressions:2 breaths (80 to 100 compressions/min) for an adult.

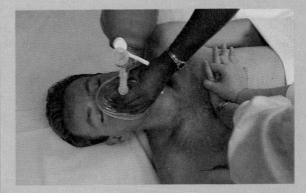

8. Continue four cycles of 15 compressions and 2 breaths, and reassess the patient's breathing and circulation.
9. Two-rescuer CPR is usually only performed in health care institutions and is not normally taught to the general public. If two rescuers are available in a health care setting, one rescuer gives chest compressions while the other performs rescue breathing. The ratio for two-rescuer CPR is 5 compressions:1 breath.

to questions, stops following directions, or suddenly becomes unconscious, call for assistance without leaving the patient. The patient's behavior may be affected by a medication or neurologic or psychotic disorder. Check the patient's chart for documentation of recently prescribed medications, nursing notes, and diagnoses that may explain the change in behavior. Be prepared to inform a nurse or physician about the time the behavior change began, the preceding events, any examinations you performed, and other pertinent information. If you are performing an examination, stop until the physician or nurse indicates you may begin again. As mentioned, never leave a patient unattended.

A patient's level of consciousness is evaluated using the **Glasgow Coma Scale** (Table 9-1). This objective numerical scale allows a patient's neurologic status to be evaluated over time; a higher score indicates a higher level of functioning.

SEIZURES

Seizures are caused by neurologic changes in brain function resulting from acute focal or generalized disturbances in the cerebrum. Patients generally lose consciousness and may exhibit convulsive movements. There are basically three types of seizures: partial (focal), petit mal (absence), and grand mal (tonic-clonic) seizures.

TABLE 9-1

GLASGOW COMA SCALE		
ACTION	**RESPONSE**	**SCORE**
Eyes open	Spontaneously	4
	To speech	3
	To pain	2
	None	1
Best verbal response	Oriented	5
	Confused	4
	Inappropriate words	3
	Incomprehensible sounds	2
	None	1
Best motor response	Obeys commands	6
	Localized pain	5
	Flexion withdrawal	4
	Abnormal flexion	3
	Abnormal extension	2
	Flaccid	1
Highest possible score		*15*

PARTIAL SEIZURES

A **partial seizure** usually begins in the hand or foot and moves up the extremity. It lasts 1 to 4 minutes, and the patient appears alert but is nonresponsive. The seizure can remain localized or can spread to other parts of the cerebrum, resulting in a loss of consciousness. A patient may be confused for 1 to 2 minutes after a partial seizure.

PETIT MAL SEIZURES

A **petit mal seizure,** which is sometimes called an *absence seizure,* occurs without warning. This type of seizure is more common during childhood and adolescence and decreases in frequency with age. A patient having a petit mal seizure abruptly stops all activity and may exhibit eye or muscle flutterings. Symptoms include a sudden loss of consciousness with eyes focusing straight ahead and a blank facial expression, cessation of motor activity, and a possible loss of muscular functioning, which may result in a fall. The patient may be totally unaware that anything has happened and may resume speaking as if they had not been interrupted; the seizure may only last 10 to 30 seconds. Petit mal seizures are not as frightening as grand mal seizures, but the momentary loss of consciousness presents safety concerns.

GRAND MAL SEIZURES

A **grand mal seizure** is typically preceded by an aura. An aura consists of symptoms such as certain smells, flashing lights, spots before the eyes, or dizziness that serve as warnings of impending seizures. Patients who are aware of this aura may seek safety and privacy before the seizure begins.

After the aura phase, a sudden contraction of thoracic and abdominal muscles forces air through the glottis causing the patient to cry out. Immediately after the cry the patient usually loses consciousness, often for several minutes. The patient may slump to the floor and experience convulsive arm and leg movements caused by tonic-clonic contractions of the extremities, trunk, and head muscles. Respiration may cease, and cyanosis occurs if emergency action is not taken to maintain the airway. Frequently the jaw is clenched, the eyes roll upward, and the pupils dilate. Patients may lose control of their bladders and bowels.

A grand mal seizure usually lasts 2 to 5 minutes and may be followed by a phase called the *postictal period.* Patients in this phase may go into a deep sleep or appear groggy and confused. They may also complain of headaches and muscle soreness. They may not be aware they have had a seizure. Patients often experience general fatigue for 1 to 2 days after grand mal seizures. Witnessing a grand mal seizure for the first time can be frightening.

PATIENT SAFETY DURING A SEIZURE

Regardless of the type of seizure a patient is having, the most important factor to remember is safety. If the patient is in a bed, make sure side rails are up and padded. (Pad the side rails with blankets or bedpads to prevent the patient from being injured.) A patient who is on the examination table should be watched closely and never left unattended. Be sure to document events that occur before, during, and after a seizure, including the aura (as described by the patient), the presence or absence of a cry, a description and the duration of body movements, a description of general behavior and behavior and orientation during the postictal phase, the patient's level of consciousness, any injuries sustained, and the duration of the entire seizure. See Procedure 9-4 for the care of a patient having a seizure.

FAINTING

Fainting, or **syncope,** is caused by decreased perfusion to the brain. The drop in perfusion may be caused by heart arrhythmia, vascular stenosis, orthostatic hypotension, hunger, sudden emotional shock, fatigue, or inadequate respirations. As mentioned previously, orthostatic hypotension is a sudden decrease in systolic blood pressure that occurs when a patient moves from a recumbent to a sitting or standing position. Poor health, especially in elderly patients, compounded by fasting for procedures or taking laxative preparations, increases the risk of fainting. Before asking patients to stand, carefully assess them for dizziness, nausea, and pallor. Assist them to an upright position, and wait a few moments to make sure they are stable before proceeding.

Watch for signs and symptoms indicating a patient may be about to faint. The patient may complain of dizziness, sweating, or feeling hot. Follow the steps in Procedure 9-5 when caring for a fainting patient.

When patients have an emotional shock or orthostatic hypotension, fainting may be expected. In other cases, however, fainting is unexpected and may happen suddenly. If a patient starts to collapse, place your knee behind the patient's knee, and with your arms around the shoulders, allow the patient to slump back against you, using your knee and body for support (Fig. 9-7). Gently ease the patient into a chair or onto the floor, taking care not to injure yourself or the patient.

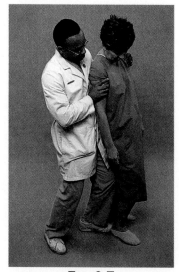

FIG. 9-7
Support of a patient who is fainting.

PROCEDURE 9-4
CARE OF A PATIENT HAVING A SEIZURE

1. Never leave the patient alone.
2. Do not try to restrain the patient during the seizure.
3. Loosen tight clothing, especially around the neck.
4. Turn the patient's head or body to one side to avoid the aspiration of excessive saliva or vomitus.
5. Do not attempt to pry the mouth open to insert a tongue blade.
6. Pad the side rails to prevent injury.
7. Provide privacy during the seizure, and keep excess noise to a minimum to avoid unnecessary stimulation that may prolong the seizure.
8. Put special mitts or tape washcloths over the patient's hands to prevent scratching.

PROCEDURE 9-5
CARE OF A FAINTING PATIENT

1. Lie the patient down.
2. Elevate the patient's feet with pillows or cushions to increase the blood flow to the brain.
3. Apply a cold cloth to the patient's forehead for comfort.
4. Watch for tachycardia, low blood pressure, pallor, and an increased respiration rate.
5. Summon a physician as soon as you have ensured the patient's safety.

SHOCK

Shock is a condition resulting from an inadequate blood flow to the peripheral tissues and vital organs. The insufficient cardiac output and maldistribution of the peripheral blood flow are not adequate for sustaining life and must be treated immediately. Types of shock include hypovolemic shock, which results from inadequate blood volume; cardiogenic shock, which results from inadequate cardiac function; vasogenic shock, which results from inadequate vasomotor tone; or a combination of these factors. Septic shock may also occur after severe bacteremia (invasion of the bloodstream by bacteria).

Common symptoms of shock include lethargy and confusion. The hands and feet may be cold, moist, and cyanotic. Also associated with shock are a weak and rapid pulse, falling blood pressure, and hyperventilation. The box summarizes the early signs and symptoms of shock.

Keep patients in shock warm, and slightly elevate their feet to improve venous blood return to the heart while you wait for a physician. If patients vomit, turn their heads to the side to prevent aspiration of the emesis. If hemorrhaging is suspected, the physician will insert a large catheter into a peripheral vein to infuse blood, fluids, and medications. The treatment for shock may include the administration of oxygen, fluids, blood, and medications to promote vasoconstriction, which elevates the blood pressure and promotes perfusion to vital organs. For severe fluid loss, such as the loss that may occur with traumatic bleeding, military antishock (MAST) trousers may be applied to redirect blood from the lower extremities to the heart, lungs, and brain. If necessary, obtain radiographs of the patient without removing the trousers.

HYPOVOLEMIC SHOCK

The most common type of shock is **hypovolemic shock.** *Hypovolemia* is defined as a decrease in circulatory blood volume. Hypovo-

---

EARLY SIGNS AND SYMPTOMS OF SHOCK

- Pallor, sweating
- Increased heart rate, respirations
- Decreased blood pressure
- Restlessness, confusion

lemia may be caused by blood or fluid loss resulting from trauma or burns, gastrointestinal bleeding, or bleeding after surgery. Patients with coagulation disorders that are vomiting excessively or have diarrhea and fluid movement into other body spaces (such as fluid movement associated with bowel obstruction) are also at risk for hypovolemic shock. The signs and symptoms of hypovolemic shock include hypotension, a weak and rapid pulse, cool and clammy skin, increased respirations, decreased urine output, and restlessness.

CARDIOGENIC SHOCK

Cardiogenic shock occurs when the heart is not able to pump an adequate volume of blood to the tissues (that is, a decrease in cardiac output). To compensate for the lower cardiac output, the heart attempts to increase its rate. The rate increase, however, may cause further damage to the heart. An increased heart rate results in less time for the coronary arteries to fill during diastole. A decrease in the perfusion of the coronary arteries with blood causes a decrease in the volume of oxygen delivered to the heart, but the heart requires more oxygen than normal because of its increased work load. Therefore an increased heart rate can both increase the heart's demand for oxygen and decrease its supply of oxygen.

The most common causes of cardiogenic shock are heart attacks, or myocardial infarctions (MIs). Other causes include pulmonary emboli, valvular disease, arrhythmias, and cardiac tamponade. Radiologic technologists frequently come in contact with patients with cardiac tamponade resulting from traumatic injuries to the chest. Blood fills the pericardium (the sac around the heart) and squeezes the heart, which interferes with its pumping ability.

VASOGENIC SHOCK

Vasogenic shock is a condition caused by massive dilation of the blood vessels and results in a rapid decrease in arterial blood pressure. Patients with cerebral trauma, sepsis, or drug intoxication are at an increased risk for shock caused by vasodilation. As the blood pressure decreases, blood pools in the vessels, and venous blood return to the heart decreases. As a result, the cardiac output decreases and the blood pressure falls even further. Patients who are in vasogenic shock caused by cerebral traumas or hemorrhages are in neurogenic shock.

Initially, patients in vasogenic shock have extremities that appear warm and pink due to the vasodilation. As the output and perfusion decrease, however, the extremities become cool and blanched.

ANAPHYLACTIC SHOCK

Anaphylactic shock is a type of vasogenic shock that occurs during severe allergic reactions. The reaction begins when histamine is released in response to antigens (foreign substances). Antigens that commonly induce anaphylaxis are insect stings, pollen, and certain drugs such as penicillin and iodinated contrast media. Histamine is a powerful vasodilator with the following effects:

1. Constriction of smooth muscle, causing bronchospasms and constriction of conducting airways (symptoms—wheezing, sneezing, and rhinitis)
2. Increased vascular permeability leading to hives (urticaria), mucosal edema (angioedema) from leakage of fluids, or red spots on the skin from leakage of blood (rash)
3. Increased mucous gland secretions (symptoms—nausea and vomiting)

Initially, a patient entering into anaphylactic shock may have hives, itching, sneezing, and a sense of apprehension. Within seconds or minutes these mild symptoms can progress to edema of the hands and face, laryngedema (wheezing respirations), dyspnea, and signs of shock (a weak and rapid pulse, falling blood pressure, and cyanosis). Unless treated immediately, the reaction may be fatal. (Drugs used to treat anaphylaxis, such as epinephrine [adrenaline], corticosteroids, and antihistamines, are discussed in Chapter 8.)

SEPTIC SHOCK

Septic shock is associated with bacteremia and a result of an inadequate supply of blood to the body tissues. Bacteremia is an invasion of the bloodstream by bacteria; it can be caused by infections after surgery or bacterial infections from IV vascular access lines or indwelling urinary catheters. Common signs of bacteremia include chills, fever, nausea, vomiting, and diarrhea.

Patients in septic shock have an increase in their heart rate and respirations, a decrease in their blood pressure and urinary output, and cool, pale, extremities. As septic shock progresses, it will result in renal failure, heart failure, respiratory insufficiency, coma, and death. Septic shock is generally treated in intensive care units with IV fluid therapy and bactericidal antibiotics.

DIABETIC EMERGENCIES

DIABETES MELLITUS

Diabetes mellitus is a chronic metabolic disorder that disrupts carbohydrate, fat, and protein metabolism and is usually related to deficient or dysfunctional insulin or to glucose intolerance. **Insulin** is a hormone secreted by the pancreas to regulate glucose levels in the body. A lack of insulin production, a deficiency in the amount of insulin, or inadequate utilization of insulin results in elevated glucose levels in the blood and glucose in the urine.

Insulin is essential for allowing the glucose in tissue cells to combine with oxygen and fuel the body. Insulin is also necessary to help the liver convert glucose to glycogen. Without insulin, glucose accumulates in the blood instead of being burned for fuel or converted to glycogen. The body must burn fat and carbohydrates simultaneously to burn fat completely. In patients with diabetes mellitus, fat is not completely metabolized, which results in the production of ketones. This condition is known as *ketosis* or *ketoacidosis*.

Diabetes mellitus has a variety of metabolic and vascular manifestations, including elevated levels of blood glucose (hyperglycemia), accelerated atherosclerosis of large vessels, microvascular disease of the retina and kidney, and demyelination and cell degeneration of the nerves (which causes neuropathy). Bacterial infections are more common in diabetics than in nondiabetics. Wounds are slow to heal and may result in ulceration and gangrene.

Type I, or insulin-dependent diabetes mellitus (IDDM), is usually diagnosed when patients are 10 to 14 years old, with boys being affected more often than girls. (IDDM was formerly known as "juvenile-onset diabetes.") Type II, or non–insulin-dependent diabetes mellitus (NIDDM), is more common (80% to 90% of all cases) and is not generally associated with ketosis.

Type II affects patients after the age of 30 and occurs more often in obese individuals, nonwhites, and females. Gestational diabetes mellitus (GDM) occurs in 20% of all pregnant women and is more likely to develop with increasing maternal age.

Patients who are required to fast for procedures should be questioned about whether they have diabetes and which types of medications they are taking. Diabetic patients who must fast should not receive food or fluid (NPO), and this should include withholding insulin until the patient is able to have food. Some physicians prefer that the patient take one half of the normal morning dose of insulin. For best results, patients who may not have anything by mouth should contact their personal physician for specific instructions.

HYPERGLYCEMIA

Hyperglycemia is an elevated blood glucose level (approximately 160 to 180 mg/ml). The glomeruli filter the glucose from the blood, but when the blood glucose level is elevated, the renal tubules are unable to resorb all the glucose and it spills into the urine. The extra glucose in the urine causes excessive urination, or **polyuria,** which in turn causes an electrolyte imbalance. The electrolyte imbalance causes an increase in serum osmolality (number of particles in the blood), which stimulates the thirst center in the hypothalamus and causes the patient to take in excessive amounts of water (referred to as **polydipsia**). Thus the classic symptoms of diabetes include pronounced thirst and frequent urination.

Hyperglycemia can cause nausea and vomiting; polyuria; polydipsia; headaches and irritability; hot, dry, and flushed skin; and hyperventilation. Hyperglycemia usually develops more slowly than hypoglycemia (an abnormally low level of glucose in the bloodstream), but if left untreated, it can become a medical emergency.

ALERT! Patients with histories of hyperglycemia should not be given glucagon for barium enema examinations because glucagon causes the blood glucose level to rise.

Stress on the body, physical or emotional, may influence the condition of a diabetic patient. Surgery, infection, and acute illness are physical stressors that may cause elevated blood glucose levels. Life changes can be emotional triggers that also cause a substantial increase in blood glucose levels. Certain medications, such as corticosteroids, diuretics, and immunosuppressive agents, may also influence blood glucose levels.

KETOACIDOSIS

Ketoacidosis results from incomplete fat metabolism. It results from a combination of abnormalities: (1) hyperglycemia, (2) acidosis, (3) low blood volume (from fluid and electrolyte loss), (4) hyperosmolality, and (5) potassium loss. Patients suffering from ketoacidosis are extremely ill and confused or comatose (in diabetic comas). Nausea and vomiting are common symptoms, as well as the classic fruity, acetone odor of the patient's breath. Insulin must be administered immediately, followed by IV fluids. In some cases, insulin may be administered in a continuous IV infusion in combination with saline. A nasogastric tube may be inserted to relieve vomiting and abdominal distention, and a urinary catheter may be required in comatose patients to monitor urine output. Most patients improve markedly within 8 hours of treatment.

HYPOGLYCEMIA

Hypoglycemia is a low blood glucose level. Hypoglycemia is a frequent complication of diabetes and is usually an effect of insulin therapy. Hypoglycemic reactions result from (1) insulin overdose, (2) inadequate food intake, (3) increased exercise, and (4) nutritional and fluid imbalances resulting from nausea and vomiting.

In the imaging department, you may encounter a patient showing the signs and symptoms of hypoglycemia, which reflect a glucose deprivation in the brain. The symptoms include cool, moist, and pale skin; confusion or behavior changes; difficulty talking; complaints of feeling weak or shaky; blurred or double vision; and an increased heart rate.

Certain medications and physical conditions unrelated to insulin may cause hypoglycemia. In addition, alcohol may cause blood glucose levels to decrease.

If patients describe any of these symptoms, assist them to a cart, monitor their vital signs frequently, and call for a physician. Hypoglycemia can lead to insulin shock. Offer the patient orange juice and hard candy or sugar. If the patient is unable to swallow, place sugar under the tongue. A bolus of 50% dextrose, an IV infusion of dextrose, or an IM injection of glucagon may also be required. The patient should be monitored carefully until the blood glucose level returns to normal and the patient's symptoms have dissipated. (Table 9-2 summarizes the management of diabetic emergencies.)

TABLE 9-2

DIABETIC EMERGENCIES

EMERGENCY	CAUSES	SIGNS	ACTION
Insulin shock (rapid onset)	Too much insulin Too little food Unusual amount of exercise Delayed meal	Excessive sweating, feeling of faintness Headache Hunger Pounding of heart, trembling, impaired vision Personality change Inability to awaken	Give the patient sugar or any food containing sugar (fruit juice, candy) Call the doctor Give glucagon if loss of consciousness occurs
Diabetic coma (slow onset)	Too little insulin Failure to follow diet Infection, fever, emotional stress	Flushed skin Increased thirst and urination Weakness, abdominal pain Loss of appetite, nausea and vomiting Coma	Call the doctor immediately Give fluids without sugar (if conscious)

SUMMARY

As a radiologic technologist, you are trained to respond to medical emergencies and should be prepared to handle unexpected situations. Be aware of the patient's level of consciousness and medical status. Be prepared to respond calmly, quickly, and appropriately to life-threatening situations. Know where emergency equipment is kept; know the way to use it, and ensure it is working properly before it is needed in a crisis situation. Become certified in CPR and maintain your certification. Develop a working knowledge of the signs and symptoms of life-threatening conditions such as shock, coma, and diabetic emergencies. Remember conditions that seem mild initially may suddenly escalate in severity and become life-threatening situations, so be prepared to respond to crisis situations without delay.

STUDY QUESTIONS

1. List the following patient conditions in order of importance:
   a. A patient is anxious about a procedure.
   b. A patient is climbing over the side rails of the stretcher.
   c. A patient becomes unresponsive; the lips and ears are cyanotic.
   d. A patient complains of chest pain.
2. Explain the technologist's role during a cardiac or respiratory arrest.
3. Describe the common signs and symptoms of respiratory distress.
4. How would you help dislodge an obstructed airway in the following patients?
   - A conscious adult
   - An unconscious adult
   - A pregnant woman
   - An infant
5. What is the ratio of chest compressions to ventilations for one-rescuer CPR? What is the ratio for two-rescuer CPR?
6. Differentiate among the three types of seizures. What should you do to assist a patient during a seizure?
7. What are the various types of shock? What are the common signs and symptoms of shock?
8. Differentiate between hyperglycemia and hypoglycemia. Which condition can lead to ketoacidosis? Which condition can lead to a diabetic coma?

Ten

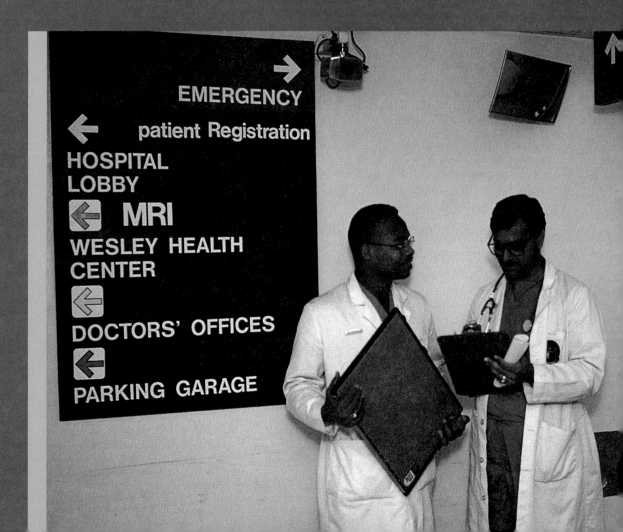

Emergency Medicine

Key Terms

Contents

Objectives

AFTER COMPLETING THIS CHAPTER, THE STUDENT WILL BE ABLE TO:

1. Identify the basic components of a well-designed emergency medical system.
2. Briefly explain the trimodal distribution of death from traumatic injuries.
3. Differentiate among the patient populations and radiologic requirements in Level I, II, and III trauma centers.
4. Describe at least three common radiologic procedures performed on trauma patients.

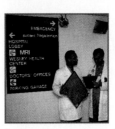

RADIOGRAPHY IS AN ESSENTIAL FUNCTION IN all emergency departments. As a radiologic technologist in an emergency department, you will encounter everything from sprained ankles to multiple trauma injuries. You must react quickly and logically when performing imaging procedures on critically ill patients who may have complex medical problems. Emergency departments are generally hectic, and you will be faced with situations not commonly encountered in other settings. Therefore having effective patient care skills is essential for performing competently and effectively in the emergency department.

EMERGENCY MEDICINE

The physicians and nurses who staff emergency departments specialize in emergency medicine. Many emergency departments also include allied health professionals such as respiratory therapists, laboratory technologists, and radiologic technologists on their staffs. In most large medical institutions a radiographic room is located within the emergency department. Smaller hospitals may transport patients to the main radiology department. In trauma cases requiring immediate performance of imaging procedures, you may have to perform mobile radiographic examinations within the trauma suite.

When patients arrive in the emergency department, they are triaged by nurses to determine their treatment priority. Patients with critical conditions are normally treated before those with minor injuries. Because many patients in emergency departments are medically unstable, you must be alert to signs and symptoms that may signal sudden changes in their conditions; examples include difficulty in breathing, changes in pulse and blood pressure, and altered states of consciousness. Immediately call a physician or nurse if a patient's condition deteriorates while they are undergoing an imaging procedure. Be prepared to initiate cardiopulmonary resuscitation (CPR) if necessary.

Take universal precautions when coming into contact with a patient's blood or body fluids. Patients are often given radiographic examinations when they have lacerations to rule out the possibility of underlying bone fractures or locate foreign bodies within the wound. As mentioned previously, gowns, gloves, masks, and eye shields should be worn when working with trauma patients because of the high probability of coming into contact with blood or body fluids.

In the United States the most common cause of death for people under age 45 is **trauma.** The Committee on Trauma of the American College of Surgeons (ACS) has created a set of guidelines to help ensure optimal patient care for patients with serious traumatic injuries. These guidelines are periodically revised to include new information and medical treatments. Most trauma facilities follow these guidelines.

A well-designed **emergency medical system (EMS)** provides patient access, prehospital care, field **triage,** acute hospital care, and facilities designed specifically for trauma and rehabilitation. The best care for trauma patients includes capable personnel and sophisticated equipment. Therefore severely injured patients are not automatically transported to the nearest hospital if a trauma center better suits their needs.

When trauma patients are triaged, their injuries are classified as immediate (life threatening), urgent, or nonurgent. Obviously, life-threatening injuries must be addressed first. Although statistics indicate that only 5% of all trauma patients have life-threatening injuries, these types of injuries are responsible for 50% of all in-hospital trauma deaths.

Statistics show that deaths from traumatic injuries have a tri-modal distribution, meaning that most deaths occur during one of three critical periods after a trauma. The first crucial period is only seconds after an injury. Death during this period could be a result of lacerations of the brain, upper spinal cord, heart, or great vessels.

The second key period occurs during the first 4 hours after an injury. Deaths during this period usually result from intracranial hemorrhaging, lacerations of the liver or spleen, or multiple injuries with significant blood loss. This is the crucial period in which emergency department treatment plays an important role.

The third period occurs during the days or weeks following the traumatic event. Deaths during this period usually result from infection or multiple organ failure.

TRAUMA CENTERS

In the past, trauma victims were usually rushed to the closest available hospitals for treatment. Because specialized treatment is needed for trauma patients, this approach is no longer acceptable. Today, medical facilities are designated as level I, level II, or level III facilities, and trauma patients are transported to the most appropriate facility for their individual needs.

Each facility plays an important role in the trauma system and must evaluate its resources. Ideally, the capabilities of a hospital and its personnel are sufficient to accommodate the severity of a transported trauma patient's injuries; this improves patient care, increases efficiency, and lowers the cost in both dollars and lives.

LEVEL I MEDICAL FACILITIES

A **level I trauma center** is the primary hospital in a trauma system. It provides total care for all injuries. Level I hospitals are generally large medical institutions that serve as both acute- and tertiary-care hospitals. Specialized medical personnel, equipment, and facilities are available in level I trauma centers as well as rapid intrahospital transportation systems.

Radiology personnel and equipment requirements include 24-hour, in-house coverage by a radiologic technologist who can perform emergency radiographic, surgical radiographic, fluoroscopic, and computed tomographic procedures. In addition, a level I hospital must be able to perform angiographies, sonographies, nuclear medicine studies, and neuroradiology procedures as needed.

LEVEL II MEDICAL FACILITIES

The most prevalent trauma facilities are **level II trauma centers.** These hospitals serve as community trauma centers, transporting patients to level I facilities only when necessary.

Radiology personnel and equipment requirements include 24-hour, in-house coverage by a radiologic technologist who can perform emergency radiographic, surgical radiographic, and fluoroscopic procedures. Level II hospitals must also be able to perform angiographic and computed tomographic procedures as needed.

LEVEL III MEDICAL FACILITIES

Level III trauma centers are generally located in rural areas and serve communities that do not have level II facilities. Level III hospitals generally have radiologic technologists and other health care professionals on call.

TRAUMA PROTOCOLS

RADIOGRAPHY OF THE CHEST

Because every trauma patient is triaged in the emergency department, the most critical and life-threatening injuries are treated first.

1. List the necessary components of a well-designed emergency medical system.
2. Explain the trimodal distribution of death from traumatic injury, and give one example of a type of death that may occur in each period.
3. On which trauma center level is the primary hospital in the trauma system?
4. Which radiologic personnel must be available on a 24-hour basis for level I and II trauma centers?
5. List four common radiologic procedures performed on trauma patients. Which procedure is performed first on patients with spinal traumas?

Eleven

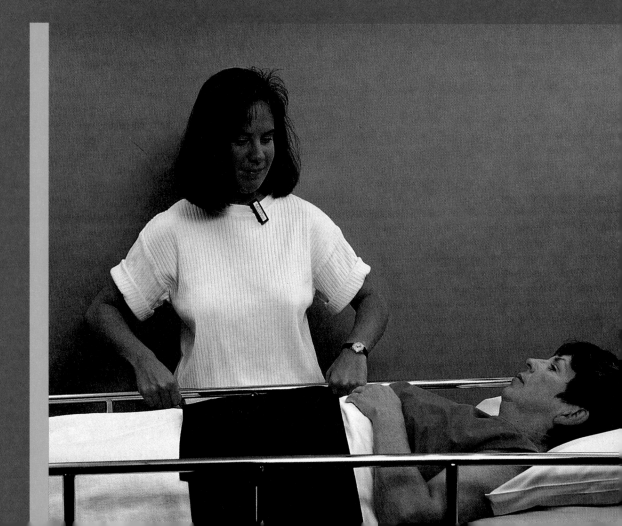

Safety

Key Terms

Contents

Objectives

AFTER COMPLETING THIS CHAPTER, THE STUDENT WILL BE ABLE TO:

1. Demonstrate transfer techniques, the use of safety devices for transporting patients on carts and wheelchairs, and other safety measures to prevent falls.
2. Explain the concept of emergency preparedness and demonstrate the way to respond to possible disasters.
3. Follow the mechanical and electrical safety procedures of the imaging department.

4. Describe the components of a hazardous communication program and explain the importance of material safety data sheets.
5. Take steps to prevent fires and react quickly and appropriately to fires.
6. Demonstrate proper radiation safety practices.
7. List the cardinal principles of radiation protection.

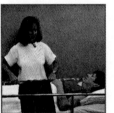 SAFETY IS IMPORTANT IN ALL HEALTH CARE settings. Everyone working in or visiting your health care facility should follow safety procedures. Safety procedures ensure that your imaging department remains a safe environment for patients, visitors, and employees.

Creating a safe environment involves addressing several key areas, including patient-fall prevention, emergency preparations, mechanical and electrical safety, safe use of hazardous materials, and fire safety. General safety guidelines are listed in the box.

In addition to the safety steps you and other staff members take, environmental safety inspections should be conducted periodically in your facility to ensure safe conditions and operating procedures. Any hazards found during inspections should be addressed promptly.

GENERAL SAFETY GUIDELINES

Walk, don't run.

Obey all warning signs, tags, and notices.

Move cautiously when pushing objects, especially when approaching blind corners.

Do not obstruct your vision with objects while carrying or pushing them.

Never use your hands to compress trash in a trash container.

Clean spilled liquids on floors and around equipment as soon as possible to avoid slips and falls. Follow material safety data sheet guidelines when cleaning chemicals and potentially hazardous material spills.

Take extra precautions when using any chemical around a patient. Be careful with hot beverages that can spill and burn patients.

Use locks and follow the principles of good body mechanics when transporting patients from carts and wheelchairs to imaging tables.

Never leave a patient unattended on a radiographic table.

Keep floors and hallways unobstructed, and always return equipment and supplies to their proper places after use.

PREVENTING PATIENT FALLS

Patient falls comprise a third of all dangerous incidents in most medical facilities. The most common patient falls occur when patients are moving or being moved from one place to another. Falls can cause broken bones and other serious injuries. Protect patients from falls by following the guidelines listed in the box.

EMERGENCY PREPAREDNESS

All medical facilities and imaging departments have policies and procedures regarding weather alerts, bomb threats, and disaster plans. You must become familiar with **emergency preparedness** plans in your own facility before an emergency occurs so that if one arises, you can react quickly and efficiently.

WEATHER ALERTS

Tornado and hurricane alerts may require you to take emergency action to ensure the safety of you and your patients. Weather alerts are usually announced over a facility's paging system. Move all patients and staff to safe areas away from windows. Some institutions may require you to secure imaging equipment to avoid damage to or injury from the equipment if it falls or breaks.

GUIDELINES FOR PREVENTING FALLS

When transporting patients, secure them with seat belts and make sure cart rails are up (Fig. 11-1).

When transferring patients into and out of wheelchairs or carts, always lock the wheels.

Assist patients in and out of wheelchairs. Move leg and foot rests out of the way.

Assist patients from carts to radiographic tables and back as described in Chapter 6.

Escort ambulatory patients in hallways, and help them onto and off tables.

Explain to patients the way in which you will assist them before moving them, and if possible, enlist their help.

If necessary, ask another staff person to help you move or position a patient safely.

Ensure that all patients wear slippers or shoes to prevent slips and falls.

When performing portable imaging procedures, return the patient's bed rails to the upright position before leaving the room.

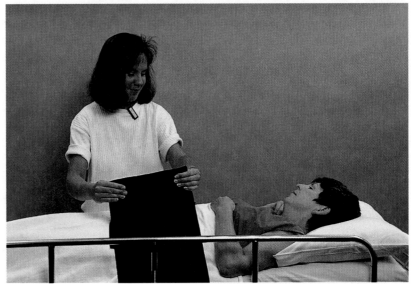

FIG. 11-1 Secure patients and raise side rails whenever transporting them.

BOMB THREATS

If you receive a telephone call in which a person makes a bomb threat, try to keep the caller on the telephone as long as possible. Take note of any distinguishing voice characteristics. Pay attention to the pitch of the caller's voice and any accent, slurring of words, or stuttering. Note any background noises such as cars, sirens, motors, paging systems, other voices, chimes, and bells. If possible, try to get the caller to tell you where the bomb is and the time at which it is set to go off. Also try to determine whether the caller seems familiar with your facility. Immediately after the person has ended the call, contact hospital security department personnel and follow their directions.

If you find a suspicious package, *do not open or touch it*. Keep patients, visitors, and personnel away, and report the package immediately.

DISASTER PLAN

Most imaging departments have a working **disaster plan** for dealing with victims of major disasters, such as those involved in airplane crashes, major industrial accidents, or explosions. A disaster would probably require you to perform additional duties. You might be asked to help transport patients or care for victims.

Portable radiographic equipment may be used in various locations in the facility to help ensure timely treatment.

Become familiar with your institution's disaster policies and procedures. In addition, most institutions hold disaster drills yearly (or more often) to ensure quick responses to actual disasters. Written disaster plans are usually found in department or facility policy or procedure manuals.

MECHANICAL AND ELECTRICAL SAFETY

Electricity can be a danger to everyone in a medical facility. Imaging departments have several pieces of electrical equipment, ranging from items as large as radiographic units to items as small as cardiac monitors. All mechanical and electrical equipment must function properly and safely. Visually inspect each piece of equipment periodically. Check x-ray tubes, hangers, tables, generators, and all other equipment used during radiographic procedures and life-saving maneuvers. Immediately report any hazardous conditions to prevent accidents.

You must also report information that suggests a piece of equipment may not be operating normally. Report situations in which a device has been dropped, a piece of equipment smells or feels warm and may have overheated, a device is unusually noisy, or a power cord is frayed or worn. Electrical incidents that should always be reported include a person being electrically shocked or the malfunctioning of a piece of equipment.

Be familiar with each room in which you work, and know where the main power switch and breaker control panels are located. In emergencies, you must be able to react quickly and turn off the main power source (Fig. 11-2).

Take the precautions listed in the box to ensure the safety of both staff and patients. Following these simple directions and being alert to possible hazards greatly reduces the chance of electrical and mechanical accidents occurring in your imaging department.

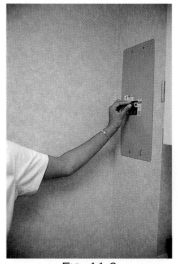

FIG. 11-2
Turn off the main power switch in an electrical emergency.

MEDICAL DEVICE REPORTING

As mentioned, you must report any unusual incident that occurs with a medical device to supervisory personnel. Medical devices are federally regulated by the Food and Drug Administration (FDA) and are covered under the Federal Food, Drug, and Cosmetic Act. **Medical device reporting** legislation requires institutions to report all malfunctions to ensure they are corrected and prevent or

ELECTRICAL SAFETY GUIDELINES

Never attempt to repair an electrical device.

Never disconnect an electrical plug from the wall by pulling on its cord. Instead, grasp the actual plug to remove it from the outlet.

Do not use multiple outlet adapters and extension cords unless they have been approved by the biomedical engineering or maintenance department. Use three-pronged plugs and outlets.

Avoid contact with water when working with electrical devices. Watch for any spills on the floor, and be sure your hands are dry. Be very careful when cleaning equipment, and always follow the manufacturer's cleaning guidelines.

Do not use any equipment with frayed or kinked cords.

Keep electrical cords out of doorways and walkways.

minimize further malfunctions. Each medical facility must have an organization-wide system for documenting, reviewing, and reporting medical device incidents. In unusual incidents, you may be asked to provide the following information:

1. Device-identifier information such as the manufacturer name, brand name, model number, and serial number
2. Device maintenance and service information
3. Pertinent patient information
4. Specific information about the unusual event

HAZARDOUS MATERIALS

Employees have a right to know about the hazards associated with chemicals used within a facility. Chemicals in the imaging department include cleaning agents and film-processing chemicals. Health care facilities must follow the **hazardous communications** rules established by the Occupational Safety and Health Administration (OSHA).

Companies that supply chemicals are responsible for informing facilities of the associated dangers of working with the chemicals. This information is supplied on a material safety data sheet (MSDS), which should accompany each chemical (Fig. 11-3). The imaging department must also clearly label chemical containers to identify their contents and display any warnings about the chemicals.

Colored triangles are commonly used to identify chemical containers. The left (blue) section of the triangle represents health; the

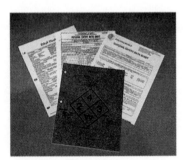

FIG. 11-3
Material safety data sheets (MSDS).

top (red) section, flammability; and the right (yellow) section, reactivity. Each section is numbered from 0 to 4, with 1 designating a low hazard and 4 designating an extreme hazard.

In addition to labeling containers, all employees must be given information and training about chemicals they use, including problems the chemicals can cause if not handled properly, emergency procedures, proper disposal, and clean-up procedures for spills. OSHA requires annual employee training on chemical hazards.

Chemicals and other substances used in facilities should be kept in their original containers with appropriate labels and should never be moved into unmarked (or any other) containers. Do not use any substance in an incorrectly labeled container, even if you think you know its contents.

MATERIAL SAFETY DATA SHEETS

A **material safety data sheet** must be available to all employees for each chemical used in the work area. It must be easily accessible and contain the following information:
1. Material identification
2. Ingredients and hazards
3. Physical data
4. Fire and explosion hazards
5. Reactivity data
6. Health hazards
7. Spill, leak, and disposal procedures
8. Special protection information
9. Special precautions and comments

The material identification section includes the name of the chemical and any other names by which it is known, in addition to the name and address of its manufacturer. The ingredients section lists the concentration percentages of the chemical's ingredients and possibly additional information. The physical data section describes the appearance, odor, boiling point, molecular weight, specific gravity, and solubility of the chemical. The fire and explosion section includes the chemical's flash point, method of ignition, and its flammability limits in air. It also describes the proper method for extinguishing a fire involving the chemical. The reactivity section lists all reagents and materials incompatible with the chemical and describes the reaction that occurs when they are mixed. The health-hazard section explains the way the chemical enters the body, its effects on the body, and first aid treatments. The spill section describes the proper procedures for the clean up and disposal of the chemical. The special protection section specifies the safety apparel, such as goggles, gloves, and gowns, that should be worn when working with the chemical. This section also describes the safety equipment, such as fire extinguishers and eye wash stations, that should be accessible when working with the chemical. The special precautions section provides information about the proper storage and handling of the chemical.

FIRE SAFETY

Fire safety starts with prevention (box). Being prepared to react to a fire is critical in health care facilities. Many patients cannot evacuate their areas without assistance, so you must be prepared to act quickly if your facility has a fire. First, you should know the exact location of your fire alarm pull station and closest fire extinguisher (Figs. 11-4 and 11-5), in addition to being familiar with the different types of fire extinguishers (box) and knowing the way to operate them.

If a fire occurs in your imaging department, you must move anyone who is in immediate danger out of the area. People who are close to fires, even small ones, are in danger and should be evacu-

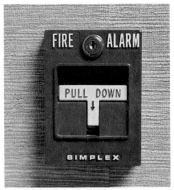

FIG. 11-4
Know the location of the nearest fire alarm.

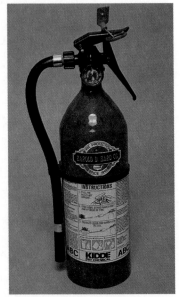

FIG. 11-5
Fire extinguisher.

GUIDELINES FOR FIRE PREVENTION

Because many fires are caused by electrical problems, always follow the previously mentioned guidelines for electrical safety.

Only allow smoking in designated areas. Be aware of patients who may try to "sneak a smoke" in unsafe areas.

When oxygen is in use, prevent the generation of flames and sparks from electrical equipment.

Use extreme care when working with flammable liquids. Store them properly and follow the special procedures for disposing of rags and cloths used with flammable liquids.

TYPES OF FIRE EXTINGUISHERS

TYPE A: For paper and rubbish fires

TYPE B: For grease and anesthetic gas fires

TYPE C: For electrical fires

ated. Turn off electrical equipment and any oxygen in use. Pull the fire alarm closest to the fire, and call the operator or safety or security department, which alerts necessary personnel and the fire department.

When all patients and visitors have been moved to safe locations and the proper authorities have been notified, contain the fire. Close windows and doors, including stairwell barrier doors, and clear corridors and exits. Finally, if you can do so safely, try to extinguish the fire with the proper type of fire extinguisher, but do not put yourself at risk. If you cannot safely extinguish the fire, move to a safe location and wait for the fire department. The box summarizes the fire emergency procedures, known as the **RACE guidelines.**

RADIATION SAFETY

In most areas of medical imaging, some type of radiation is used in imaging procedures on the body. Ionizing radiation (the radiation produced in x-ray examinations) ionizes atoms in the body. Atoms in the body normally exist in a neutral state, but when struck by the energy of an x-ray, atoms can assume positive charges (and become cations) or negative charges (and become anions). Thus, x-rays are classified as sources of ionizing radiation.

UNITS OF RADIATION MEASUREMENT

The field of radiology uses specific terms to describe units of radiation. Be familiar with the most common units of measurement. The **roentgen (R)** is the unit used for measuring radiation exposure in air and defining radiation quantities and intensities. The **rad** is the radiation absorbed dose. A rad differs from a roentgen in that it takes the biologic effects of the type of radiation a patient has been exposed to into consideration. The rad is commonly used to

---

IN A FIRE EMERGENCY, REMEMBER TO RACE:

R **R**emove and **R**escue all individuals in immediate danger
A **A**lert the proper authorities by **A**ctivating the pull station **A**larm and **A**nnouncing the fire
C **C**ontain the fire by **C**losing doors
E **E**xtinguish the fire with the proper type of **E**xtinguisher

describe the amount of radiation that has been received by a patient. With modern radiologic equipment, patient radiation doses are relatively small. Therefore you will usually encounter exposure values measured in millirads (mrads); 1 mrad = $^1/_{1000}$ rad.

Another unit, the **rem,** represents the quantity of radiation received by those working with radiation. Rem stands for "rad equivalent man"; it is used when reporting the radiation exposure of personnel monitoring devices. Like the rad, the rem factors in the biologic effects of the specific type of radiation to which the person is exposed. Again, because the amounts of radiation most personnel are exposed to are relatively small, personnel monitoring reports are measured in mrem.

RADIATION PROTECTION

Although in-depth discussions of radiation safety and physics are beyond the scope of this text, the cardinal principles of radiation protection are reviewed here. Safe radiation practices are vital for protecting you and your patients from exposure. You can minimize radiation exposure in the three following ways:

1. Minimize the time you are exposed to ionizing radiation.
2. Maximize the distance between the radiation source and the individual being exposed.
3. Maximize the amount of shielding material between the radiation source and the individual being exposed.

Radiation exposures for patients and technologists should always be *a*s *l*ow *a*s *r*easonably *a*chievable (**ALARA**). Avoid unnecessary radiation exposure. Do not stay in a room during an exposure unless it is absolutely necessary. When performing fluoroscopic procedures, wear appropriate protective apparel such as lead aprons and gloves. Use gonadal shields on all patients when possible, and perform radiologic procedures accurately to prevent repeat examinations. Remember that although the information gained from radiologic examinations is vital for quality patient care, radiologic procedures must be conducted using the lowest possible doses of radiation. This is primarily a responsibility of radiologic technologists because they control the x-ray equipment operations.

SUMMARY

Protection and safety are basic necessities. You can protect patients and yourself by ensuring your environment is safe. A safe environment reduces the risks of accidents and illnesses. Know the locations of emergency exits, fire alarm pull stations, and fire extinguishers. Know the location of the main circuit breakers so that you can turn off the power supply in an emergency if necessary. Have a working knowledge of your institution's disaster plan, and be prepared to respond to crisis situations. Handle equipment and supplies safely and be attentive to possible safety hazards.

STUDY QUESTIONS

1. Describe at least four general safety guidelines to follow in all medical facilities. For what reasons are these important?
2. Describe a common cause of patient falls in imaging departments. In what way can this be avoided?
3. Explain the procedure to follow if you receive a telephone call in which a person makes a bomb threat.
4. What is a disaster plan and why is it necessary?
5. Specify three electrical and mechanical situations that should be reported to maintain safety.
6. Briefly describe the nine elements of a material safety data sheet.
7. Explain the fire procedures represented by the acronym RACE.
8. List the three types of fire extinguishers and their uses.
9. Differentiate among the roentgen, rad, and rem units of radiation measurement.
10. Explain the three cardinal principles of radiation protection.

Twelve

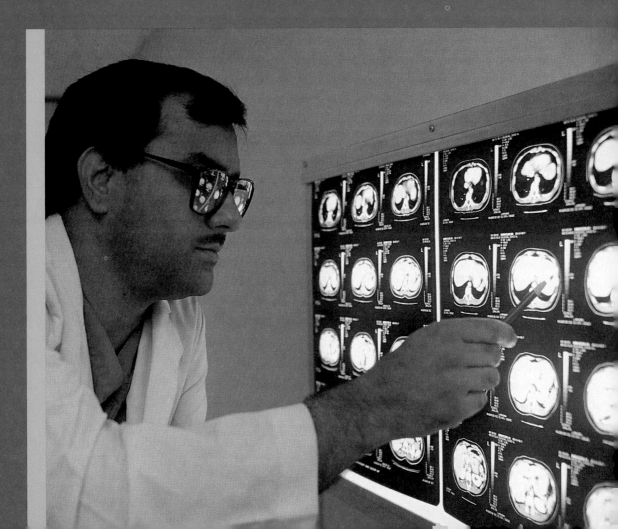

Patient Care in Specialty Areas

Key Terms

Contents

Objectives

AFTER COMPLETING THIS CHAPTER, THE STUDENT WILL BE ABLE TO:

1. Explain the role mammography plays in diagnosing and treating breast disease.
2. Document proper health histories for mammographic evaluations.
3. Explain the difference in the way images are produced with conventional radiographic and computed tomographic examinations.
4. Identify the types of contrast agents used in computed tomographic imaging and the importance of adequate patient preparation.
5. Describe procedures commonly performed in the angiography suite.
6. List the risks of an arteriogram.
7. Describe the basic components of an electrocardiogram.
8. Identify life-threatening dysrhythmias.
9. List the signs and symptoms of bleeding associated with biopsies.
10. Compare conventional radiography with diagnostic medical sonography.
11. List three body parts that may be examined with ultrasound imaging.
12. Demonstrate the proper care and handling of the transducers used in ultrasound.
13. Compare conventional radiographic imaging to magnetic resonance imaging.
14. List three body parts that may be examined with magnetic resonance imaging.
15. Document proper histories and screenings of patients entering the magnet room.
16. Identify contraindications to magnetic resonance examinations.
17. Compare radiographic imaging with nuclear medicine studies.
18. Briefly explain the reason radiopharmaceuticals are used in nuclear medicine imaging.

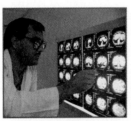

AS AN IMAGING PROFESSIONAL, YOU MAY perform procedures beyond general radiographic and fluoroscopic examinations. As discussed in Chapter 1, several of these modalities may be learned on the job. Some modalities, such as mammography, computed tomography (CT), cardiovascular-interventional procedures, and nuclear medicine studies, use ionizing radiation. A few modalities, such as ultrasound and magnetic resonance imaging (MRI), use nonionizing radiation.

In all instances, communication skills appropriate for individual patients are essential. All patients must be kept safe, secure, and comfortable, and their care kept confidential. General patient care issues such as infection control, patient assessment and assistance, and medication administration are components of all clinical situations. This chapter describes key features and patient-care issues relevant to each of the various imaging modalities.

MAMMOGRAPHY

The specialized field known as **mammography** centers around radiography of the breast. Mammography uses radiologic equipment manufactured specifically for breast imaging (Fig. 12-1). Low-energy x-rays are used in conjunction with film and screen combinations designed for exceptional visualization of the soft tissues of the breast.

Mammography has an important role in the screening, detection, and treatment of breast cancer. The American Cancer Society recommends that women from 35 to 40 years of age have baseline mammograms, women from 40 to 50 years of age have a mammogram every 2 years, and women more than 50 years of age have an annual mammogram. When combined with physical breast examinations, mammography is the best method available to detect breast cancer in its early stages. The earlier breast cancer is detected, the better the woman's chance of survival.

Mammography can be used to screen asymptomatic women or evaluate palpable breast masses in both women and men (Fig. 12-2). When a mass is identified, mammography can localize the mass for a surgical or core-needle biopsy for pathologic evaluation. During a core-needle biopsy, samples of tissue are taken from in and around the lump using specialized, large-bore needles. The tissue samples are examined carefully by a pathologist to determine the cause of the mass.

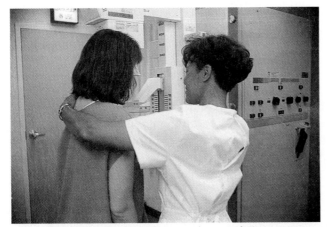

FIG. 12-1 Maintain patient dignity and respect during a mammographic examination.

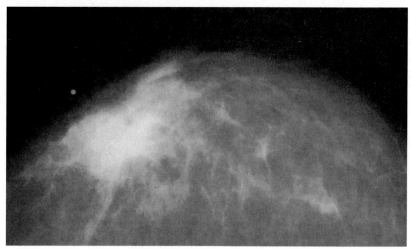

FIG. 12-2 A mammographic image of the breast.

The Food and Drug Administration (FDA) closely monitors and regulates mammography to ensure the highest-quality patient care and has recently developed the Mammography Quality Standard Act (MQSA). The MQSA regulates the equipment, quality-assurance testing, and qualifications of mammographers and radiologists involved in mammography. Mammographers are required to maintain automatic processors, darkrooms, film and cassettes, and mammographic equipment in compliance with strict quality control standards. Both mammographers and radiologists must fulfill continuing education requirements and routinely conduct quality assurance studies, such as comparison of pathologic evaluation of breast masses with radiologic findings to assist in monitoring competence and job knowledge. Ensure that patients receive necessary follow-up information when radiographic findings suggest abnormalities in breast tissue.

BREAST CANCER AWARENESS AND EDUCATION

Patient rapport and excellent communication (as described in Chapter 2) are essential components in quality mammographic examinations. Carefully explain mammographic procedures to patients and answer any questions they may have regarding examinations and their possible outcomes. Effective communication skills can help ease patients' fears and apprehensions. Preserve patients' privacy and dignity throughout the examinations. Many breast imaging centers also educate women about breast self-examinations (BSEs). Mammographers must be well educated about diseases of the breast in addition to breast imaging because they often serve as educators on a wide range of topics in mammography.

Breast tissue must be compressed during radiographic exposures to obtain high-quality images. For many patients, this compression is painful. Explain the importance of good compression in producing quality diagnostic images while remaining empathetic to each patient's needs. Carefully explain the procedure in advance, and listen carefully to patients' concerns and questions.

MAMMOGRAPHY HEALTH HISTORY DOCUMENTATION

The exact cause of breast cancer is unknown, but it is believed to be caused by a number of factors. Record and maintain a complete medical history for each person receiving a mammogram (Fig. 12-3). Include information about the woman's family health history as well as her own because heredity, endocrine disorders, dietary habits, and oncogenic and environmental factors may contribute to the risk of developing breast cancer.

COMPUTED TOMOGRAPHY

Computed tomography (CT) provides sectional images of the body. CT equipment includes a specialized x-ray tube and detectors located within the gantry of the CT unit (Fig. 12-4). A computer analyzes the x-ray information and produces the images. Each image is composed of many elements called **pixels.** The pixels are displayed in rows and columns and form a **matrix.** Images produced by computers are known as *digital images.* Images can be processed in a variety of body planes for final interpretation. They may be displayed on computers or printed as hard copies for interpretation.

CT can reveal small variances in tissue densities (Fig. 12-5) more effectively than conventional radiographic imaging. CT is used to image various body parts and can detect soft tissue masses, cysts, aneurysms of the aorta and brain, intracerebral hemorrhages, abnormal fluid collections such as abscesses, and some spinal abnormalities such as disk herniations. CT is often used in combination with conventional radiography to diagnose and treat disease.

PATIENT PREPARATION FOR COMPUTED TOMOGRAPHIC EXAMINATIONS

Most CT examinations require the use of contrast agents to aid in the diagnosis of abnormalities. Before giving patients contrast media, ask patients whether they have had allergic reactions after pre-

Ohio State University Mammography

SSN: _____ MEDICAL RECORD #: _____ DATE OF MAMMOGRAM: ___/___/___

NAME: _____ _____ MAIDEN NAME: _____ AGE: _____ D.O. B. ___/___/___

ADDRESS: _____ CITY: _____ STATE: _____ ZIP CODE: _____

HOME TELEPHONE: (___) _____ WORK TELEPHONE: (___) _____

PLACE OF BIRTH (CITY & STATE): _____

REFERRING PHYSICIAN: _____ PHYSICIAN'S PHONE _____

HISTORY   Reason patient referred for mammogram:

☐ ROUTINE MAMMOGRAM (PATIENT ASYMPTOMATIC)

☐ FOLLOW-UP FOR _____

☐ PATIENT SYMPTOMATIC (lump, burning, nipple discharge, nipple inversion, tenderness)

_____

_____

PERSONAL HISTORY OF:

	SIDE*	YEAR	BENIGN	MALIGNANT
Aspiration	___	___	☐	☐
Biopsy	___	___	☐	☐
Biopsy	___	___	☐	☐
Lumpectomy	___	___	☐	☐
Mastectomy	___	___	☐	☐

*Right = R; Left = L; Both = B

	RIGHT	LEFT	Year(s)
Breast Implants	☐	☐	___
Radiotherapy	☐	☐	___
Chemotherapy			___
Hormone Therapy			___
Tamoxifen			___

Have you ever been diagnosed with cancer?

No ☐   Yes ☐   Type: _____

Previous mammogram?

No ☐   Yes ☐

How many?

YEAR   PLACE (Your last two mammograms)

____ _____

____ _____

Are you now taking or have you ever taken any of the following hormone medications? (Mark all that apply.)

No ☐   Yes ☐

	Age began	Total years	Currently using
Premarin (estrogen only)	___	___	☐
Provera (estrogen + progesterone)	___	___	☐
Progesterone only	___	___	☐

Reason (Mark all that apply.):

Menopause ☐   Osteoporosis ☐   Other ☐

RIGHT   LEFT

RT. LAT.   RT. MED.   LT. MED.   LT. LAT.

Nipple markers used ☐   Lump scar ends marked ☐   Mole marked ☐   Breast self-examination instruction ☐ Yes ☐ No ☐

Technologist's signature _____

FAMILY HISTORY

Family history of breast cancer?

No ☐   Yes ☐

	Yes	How many?	Age(s) at diagnosis
Mother	☐		_____
Sister(s)	☐	_____	_____
Daughter(s)	☐	_____	_____

	Paternal	Maternal	Age(s) at diagnosis
Grandmother(s)	☐	☐	_____
Aunt(s)	☐	☐	_____
Other:			
_____	☐	☐	_____

Family history of other cancer?

No ☐   Yes ☐   If yes, list relation and type of cancer

_____

_____

GYNECOLOGICAL HISTORY

Date of last menstrual period: ____ / ____ / ____

Age at first menstrual period: ____ / ____ / ____

Have you ever had a full-term pregnancy?

No ☐   Yes ☐

Age at first full-term pregnancy: _____

Total number of live-born children: _____

Total number of children breast-fed: _____

Are you pregnant now?   No ☐   Yes ☐

Did you take DES (Diethylstilbestrol) during a pregnancy?

No ☐   Yes ☐   Unknown ☐

Did your mother take DES during her pregnancy with you?

No ☐   Yes ☐   Unknown ☐

Have you had a hysterectomy?

No ☐   Yes ☐

Age at hysterectomy _____

Type: ☐ Uterine only   ☐ Ovarian only

☐ Uterine and ovarian

☐ Not sure

Have you gone through menopause?

No ☐   Yes ☐   Currently ☐   Induced ☐

Age at menopause   _____

Are you using or have you ever used birth control pills?

No ☐   Yes ☐   Currently using

Age began   _____

Total years   _____

Height: _____ ft. _____ in.

Current weight: _____ lbs. _____   **Weight, age 18:** _____ lbs.

INFORMED CONSENT: Mammography is only one component of a complete breast evaluation. Monthly breast self-examination, regular physical examination, and regular mammography provide the most thorough evaluation available today. I give my consent for mammography. If my mammogram is abnormal, further consultation and evaluation by my physician will be required. I understand I may be contacted to confirm that I have completed recommended follow-up.

SIGNATURE _____ DATE: ____ / ____ / ____

FIG. 12-3 Medical history form for mammography.

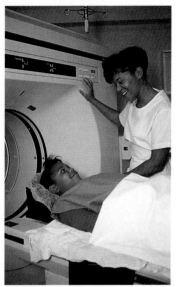

FIG. 12-4
Patients must be told to hold very
still and follow breathing instructions
during CT examinations.

vious procedures. Radiologists should be notified of previous allergic reactions. If necessary, examinations can be performed without contrast medium or after administration of medications such as cortisone or antihistamines to prevent reactions.

Intravenous (IV) iodinated contrast agents are commonly used for imaging blood vessels, identifying hemorrhages, determining the vascularity of a mass, or differentiating scar tissue from recurrent disc herniation. When contrast material is injected intravenously, patients may not have food or liquids for at least 4 hours before the procedure to reduce the risk of nausea and vomiting after injection of the iodinated contrast material.

Iodinated contrast agents or barium sulfate agents manufactured specifically for use in CT may be ingested orally or through a nasogastric tube before procedures to outline the bowel, which helps the physician distinguish bowel loops from surrounding anatomic structures in the abdomen. Before abdominal imaging procedures, patients must have bowel preps and orally ingest iodinated or barium sulfate contrast material. The contrast materials should be present in both the large and small intestines before the abdomen is

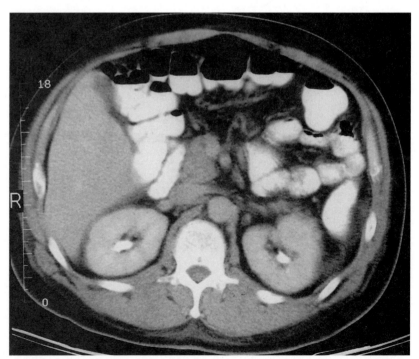

FIG. 12-5 Abdominal CT image after injection and ingestion of contrast agents.

imaged. The patient must drink the contrast material at various intervals before the examination to ensure adequate distribution of the contrast agent throughout the bowel.

Contrast media may be injected intravenously by an automatic injector to image the chest and great vessels. The bolus injection aids visualization of the vessels within the mediastinum. An IV line may be required before the procedure. Take universal precautions when starting IV lines and handling patient blood and body fluids.

CT procedures must be fully explained to all patients before their examinations. Because images must often be obtained immediately after injections, patient cooperation is critical. Although most CT procedures are performed fairly quickly and painlessly, patient motion during scans greatly degrades the quality of the final images. Patients must remain still and carefully follow breathing instructions during the scan.

COMPUTED TOMOGRAPHIC IMAGING IN INVASIVE PROCEDURES

CT may be used to guide physicians who are performing percutaneous biopsies or drainage procedures. Aspiration biopsies may be performed to withdraw fluids from a structure, and core biopsies may be performed to obtain tissue samples from masses or other abnormal structures. The biopsy samples are sent to the pathology laboratory for analysis. There are risks associated with biopsies; for example, the most common risk associated with a lung biopsy is a pneumothorax (collapse of the lung). Most biopsies also have an associated risk of infection and bleeding. Patients should be observed carefully after CT-guided invasive procedures for signs and symptoms of bleeding, pneumothorax, sepsis, and possible allergic reactions.

COMPUTED TOMOGRAPHIC IMAGING IN EMERGENCY SITUATIONS

CT is the imaging modality of choice for evaluating head traumas; it can detect life-threatening cranial bleeding (hematomas). Trauma patients' conditions are often critical and in need of immediate attention. In emergency situations, remain calm and confident. Perform procedures as expediently as possible. Patients may be combative after brain traumas, so use immobilization techniques to ensure patient safety.

New equipment allows CT scans to be obtained very quickly. Thus critically ill patients should not have to remain in the CT area for extended periods. Remember, patients should never be left unattended under any circumstances. Effective communication is always a significant part of obtaining high-quality images in all patient-care areas.

CARDIOVASCULAR-INTERVENTIONAL TECHNOLOGY

In angiography suites, patient care is often critical and complex. Patients undergoing an invasive procedure such as an angiography, a percutaneous drainage, or a percutaneous biopsy are usually quite apprehensive. Interventional procedures often require conscious sedation of the patient with special vital-sign monitoring. Drugs for conscious sedation are tailored for individual patients and can be administered as oral medications or intramuscular (IM) or IV injections. The types of IV injections range from single IV injections to continuous injections of a combination of drugs, which provide sedation throughout longer procedures. Drugs for conscious sedation have sedative effects and cause amnesia but do not cause patients to lose consciousness as general anesthesia does.

Patients are often subjected to greater risks during interventional procedures than during most other radiographic procedures. Technologists must know the possible risks and warning signs of complications. Complications include hemorrhaging or thrombosis at the catheter insertion site, infections, embolisms, and allergic reactions to contrast agents. Be alert to any bleeding, vital sign or neurologic changes, or patient complaints of pain during angiographic or invasive procedures. Hypotension and tachycardia may indicate a hemorrhage or an anaphylactic reaction to the contrast medium. A diminished peripheral pulse or altered neurologic status may indicate the formation of a thrombus or an embolus. Cardiac dysrhythmias may result from conduction disorders induced by catheters or contrast agents.

PREEXAMINATION ASSESSMENTS

To ease patients' anxieties, listen to their concerns and questions and forward them to the radiologist. Patients who understand what happens in the angiography-interventional suite and know what is expected of them during the procedure and the postprocedure recovery period are more cooperative.

Verify that the physician has obtained an informed consent (see Chapter 4). Check the patient's chart for pertinent laboratory test results such as complete blood counts (CBCs), platelet counts, prothrombin times, and electrolyte, blood urea nitrogen (BUN), and creatinine levels because abnormalities may contraindicate proceeding with an examination. Measure vital signs to provide baseline measurements for comparison with vital signs taken during and after the procedure. Ensure that the patient has had nothing to eat or drink (NPO) for 6 to 8 hours before the procedure, especially if conscious sedation drugs will be used. Take a history concentrating on allergies to medications, including preprocedure medications such as atropine, Benadryl, and sedatives. Evaluate the peripheral pulses of patients preparing to undergo angiographies, and check specific symptoms and other pertinent medical history information related to the diagnosis.

PROCEDURES

ANGIOGRAPHY

Radiography of blood or lymph vessels using iodinated contrast material is called **angiography.** This term refers to radiography of the venous, arterial, or lymph systems. The term *arteriography* refers to radiographic studies of the arteries only. The two terms are often used interchangeably.

Angiography can demonstrate narrowing in vessels (stenosis), aneurysms, arteriovenous malformations, and other vascular abnormalities. Selective catheterization of specific arteries is used to make diagnoses correlating with clinical signs and symptoms. For example, an arch aortogram with bilateral selective carotid arteriograms evaluates symptoms related to carotid stenosis. An abdominal aortogram with selective mesenteric and celiac arteriograms evaluates gastrointestinal bleeding.

The angiographic procedure begins with the percutaneous introduction of a large-bore needle into an artery, usually the femoral or brachial artery. When the needle is in the lumen of the artery, a guidewire is inserted through and then farther past the needle. The needle is withdrawn, leaving the guidewire in place. A catheter is passed over the wire into the artery. This procedure is known as the **Seldinger technique** (Fig. 12-6). At this point, the guidewire is removed and the catheter advanced to the desired site of injection or the guidewire is left in place to keep the catheter stiff while being advanced through the vascular system to a specific site. The wire is then withdrawn. The contrast agent is injected through the catheter while radiographs are taken in rapid sequence.

The risks to a patient during angiography vary according to the particular procedure used and the patient's overall health condition. Risks include but are not limited to strokes, hematomas, bleeding at

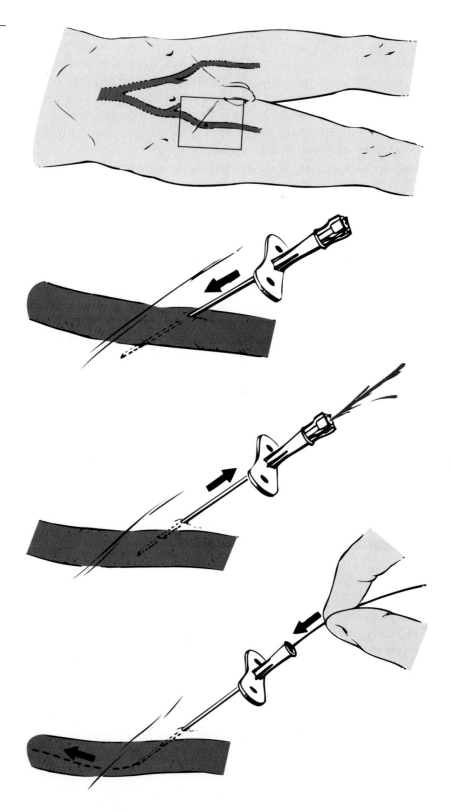

FIG. 12-6 Seldinger technique.

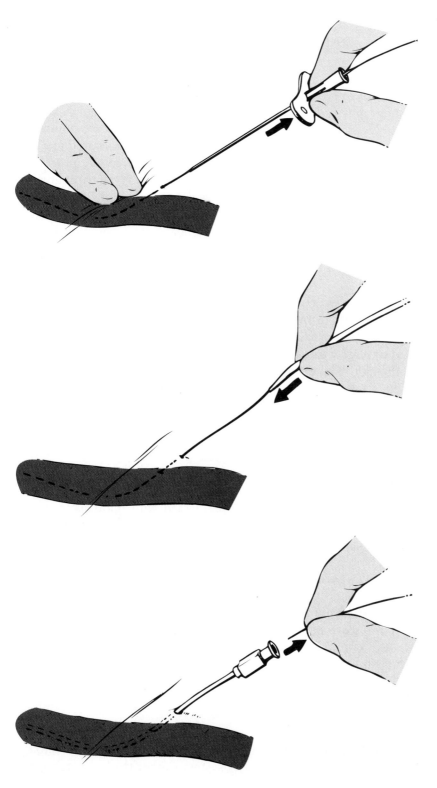

catheter sites, contrast reactions, and renal failure. As with all invasive procedures, angiography carries the risk of bleeding and infection.

ANGIOPLASTY

Angiography can visualize narrowing of an artery, which causes reduced blood flow. Some patients with this condition are candidates for **angioplasty,** in which a balloon-tipped catheter is used to dilate the narrowed portion of the vessel. This relatively safe procedure may eliminate the need for surgery. Angioplasty is not without risks, however. These risks are similar to the risks for angiography but also include tearing and puncturing of arteries, which can cause them to bleed or close suddenly. Another possible complication is a piece of plaque breaking loose and traveling to the lower part of the body, causing a decrease in circulation to the feet and toes.

THROMBOLYTIC THERAPY

Thrombolytic drugs, such as streptokinase and urokinase, may be used to dissolve acute clots in vessels. The Seldinger technique is used to place a catheter into a vein or artery and position it directly by the clot. The drug is then infused over several hours and sometimes days, with periodic angiographies through the existing catheter to recheck the vessel for patency. These types of drugs carry a considerable risk of bleeding, not only at the puncture site but elsewhere in the body. Angioplasty may be performed in conjunction with thrombolytic therapy.

BIOPSY

Percutaneous biopsies may be performed with fluoroscopic guidance. An aspiration biopsy uses a thin-walled needle inserted into an abnormal tissue (lesion) to aspirate a specimen into the needle. The specimen is placed on a slide and sent to the cytology laboratory. As discussed, a core-needle biopsy uses a large needle to remove a core or piece from the lesion; the sample is then evaluated by the pathology department.

The most common risk of a lung biopsy is a pneumothorax. Most biopsies also carry risks of infection and bleeding. Recovery time will vary according to the type of biopsy performed and other factors.

DRAINAGE

The procedure for percutaneous drainage of the biliary or urinary system is similar to that of an angiogram. A needle is placed into the biliary ducts or renal collecting system (rather than an artery), and a guidewire and catheter are threaded into the system. The catheter is left in place and drains into an external collection bag. This method may also be used to drain abscess pockets in the body.

There is a large risk of infection for patients who have invasive procedures of the urinary or biliary tract or for an abscess. Sudden chills, warm and dry flushed skin, fever, and an increase in the respiration rate all indicate the patient may have sepsis, a very serious infection from gram-negative bacteria that enter the bloodstream. Percutaneous abscess drainage, nephrostomies, and biliary drainage or stone removal can leak bacteria into the body or bloodstream. If sepsis is not treated immediately and aggressively, septic shock (vascular collapse) will develop and may lead to death. Radiologists and other physicians often treat patients undergoing invasive procedures with prophylactic antibiotics to prevent sepsis. Help minimize risks by following proper sterile-technique protocols, taking universal precautions, carefully assessing patients' conditions before and after procedures, and monitoring pertinent laboratory values.

PHYSIOLOGIC MONITORING

Electronic monitors measure and record vital signs (Fig. 12-7). Depending on the type of equipment and options included, these monitors can obtain invasive and noninvasive blood pressures, heart rates, electrocardiograph (ECG) activity, respiration rates, and oxygen saturation measurements.

To prepare patients for monitoring, you may have to attach electrodes, blood pressure cuffs, and sensors for pulse oximetry. Explain

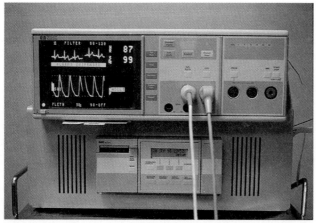

FIG. 12-7 Electronic monitor for assessing vital signs and other patient data.

to patients that although the electrical activity of the heart is being recorded, no electricity will enter their bodies.

THE ELECTROCARDIOGRAM

Only certified ECG technicians should interpret ECGs or monitor patients on ECG machines. Therefore our discussion of ECG monitoring is limited to normal and life-threatening **dysrhythmias** (abnormal rhythms) that technologists may encounter. Any abnormalities should immediately be reported to a radiology nurse or radiologist.

The ECG pattern helps reveal abnormalities that may interfere with electrical conduction in the heart. It cannot, however, reveal mechanical dysfunctioning of the myocardium. Thus a normal ECG may not necessarily indicate a patient has a normal, healthy heart.

An **electrocardiogram (ECG or EKG)** is a graphic representation of the electrical activity of the heart. Electrodes attached to patients' chests and limbs measure the impulses generated during the cardiac cycle. An image is produced in a waveform on special graph paper. Positive waveforms appear above the isoelectric line, and negative waveforms fall below. Each deflection in an ECG pattern represents a part of the cardiac cycle.

The P wave results from contraction of the atria; the QRS complex is the contraction of the ventricles. The resting stage of the atria is hidden within the QRS complex. The resting stage for the ventricles is shown by the T wave (Fig. 12-8).

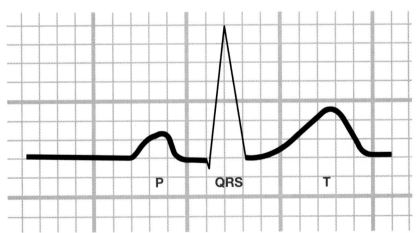

FIG. 12-8 Normal ECG waveform. (Modified from Huszar RJ, *Basic dysrhythmias: interpretation and management*, ed 2, St Louis, 1994, Mosby.)

In a normal sinus rhythm an electrical impulse originates in the sinoatrial node of the heart and follows a normal sequence of conduction. The heart rate is 60 to 100 beats/min. Fig. 12-9 shows a tracing of normal sinus rhythm that is regular and contains normal P, QRS, and T deflections.

Sinus bradycardia is a sinus rhythm, but the heart rate is below 60 beats/min (Fig. 12-10). Sinus bradycardia is the normal cardiac rhythm of some patients. Other patients with sinus bradycardia, however, require pacemakers to prevent their hearts from dropping to abnormally slow rates, which would significantly reduce cardiac output and endanger vital organs.

Sinus tachycardia is a sinus rhythm in which the heart rate ranges from 100 to 150 beats/min (Fig. 12-11). The waveform is no different from a normal waveform, except that it indicates a faster heart rate. If there is no underlying disease, sinus tachycardia may be unimportant. However, if a patient has an irritable heart, sinus tachycardia may lead to potentially life-threatening ventricular tachycardia.

A **premature ventricular contraction** or PVC is a single ectopic beat that interrupts the underlying cardiac rhythm. It is char-

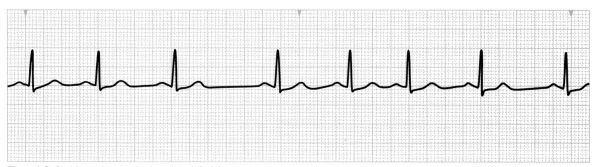

FIG. 12-9 Normal sinus rhythm. (Modified from Huszar RJ, *Basic dysrhythmias: interpretation and management*, ed 2, St Louis, 1994, Mosby.)

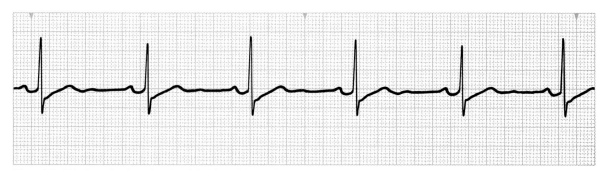

FIG. 12-10 Sinus bradycardia. (Modified from Huszar RJ, *Basic dysrhythmias: interpretation and management*, ed 2, St Louis, 1994, Mosby.)

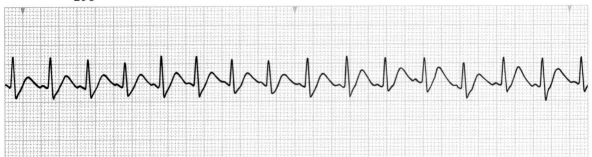

FIG. 12-11 Sinus tachycardia. (Modified from Huszar RJ, *Basic dysrhythmias: interpretation and management*, ed 2, St Louis, 1994, Mosby.)

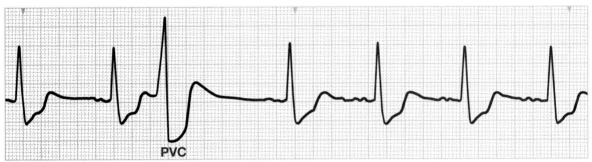

FIG. 12-12 Premature ventricular contractions. (Modified from Huszar RJ, *Basic dysrhythmias: interpretation and management*, ed 2, St Louis, 1994, Mosby.)

acterized by a wide, irregular QRS complex that has no associated P wave (Fig. 12-12). A PVC can have a positive or negative deflection or both (multifocal PVC).

Occasionally a patient undergoing a cardiac catheterization or pulmonary angiogram has PVCs resulting from the manipulation of the catheter through the heart valves. The PVCs usually cease after the manipulation ends. If the patient experiences a fluttering sensation in the chest, notify the radiologist immediately. Watch the patient closely and provide reassurance that the fluttering will soon subside. If it does not subside, you must take immediate emergency action to prevent damage to the heart. PVCs decrease cardiac output by 12% to 15% if left untreated. The most common treatment for PVCs is a lidocaine bolus followed by a lidocaine drip infusion. PVCs may progress to ventricular tachycardia or ventricular fibrillation, both of which are life-threatening heart-rhythm abnormalities.

Ventricular tachycardia (V-tach) (Fig. 12-13) is a condition in which more than six PVCs appear in a row on an ECG tracing. Although the rate is usually regular, it can be anywhere from 150 to

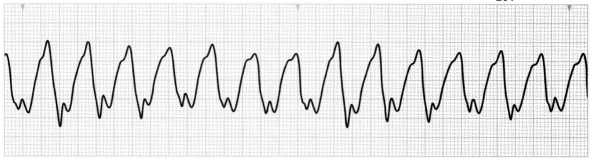

FIG. 12-13 Ventricular tachycardia. (Modified from Huszar RJ, *Basic dysrhythmias: interpretation and management*, ed 2, Mosby Lifeline, 1994.)

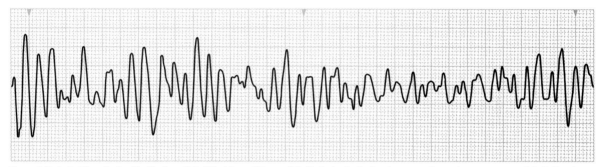

FIG. 12-14 Ventricular fibrillation. (Modified from Huszar RJ, *Basic dysrhythmias: interpretation and management*, ed 2, St Louis, 1994, Mosby.)

250 beats/min. Because the heart is beating so rapidly, cardiac output is very low. V-tach may be transient or may continue until the underlying cause is treated. The V-tach rhythm is life threatening and requires immediate intervention. The most common treatment is a lidocaine bolus administered intravenously followed by a continuous drip; in some cases, defibrillation may be necessary. The patient may lose consciousness and become hypotensive. Untreated, V-tach usually progresses to ventricular fibrillation.

Ventricular fibrillation (V-fib) is the most serious cardiac dysrhythmia a patient can have (Fig. 12-14). The ventricles are repeatedly stimulated by ectopic foci and thus generate uncoordinated, chaotic impulses, causing the heart to fibrillate rather than contract. Essentially, the heart simply quivers; there is no cardiac output. On the ECG tracing, no waves or complexes can be analyzed. V-fib is the most common cause of sudden death. Patients must be defibrillated immediately if they are to have any chance for survival.

On an ECG tracing, **asystole** (Fig. 12-15) is shown by a straight line with no deflections whatsoever, signifying that all electrical ac-

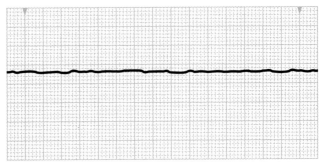

FIG. 12-15 Asystole. (Modified from Huszar RJ, *Basic dysrhythmias: interpretation and management*, ed 2, St Louis, 1994, Mosby.)

tivity in the heart has stopped. Without immediate intervention such as cardiopulmonary resuscitation (CPR), the patient will die.

When electrocardiography is being performed to identify a dysrhythmia, every lead should be checked by a technologist or nurse and all electrodes secured to the patient. If an electrode comes off a patient, there will be a flat line on the ECG. If patients move, especially their arms or legs, they may generate abnormal ECG waves similar to PVCs. Always check the patient and electrocardiograph connections when a dysrhythmia is suspected.

Make sure the patient's skin is dry when attaching electrode patches for an ECG. Use a dry gauze sponge to dry and slightly abrade the skin at the selected site, which increases the skin's contact with the electrode and creates better signal transmission. Avoid connecting electrodes to skin with a lot of hair because the patches will not adhere well. (It may be necessary to shave hair to make a connection.) Attach an electrode to each side of the chest at the level of the second intercostal space. Attach a third patch to the left lower side of the chest at the level of the sixth or seventh intercostal space. The leads are color coded and should be attached to the electrodes as shown in Fig. 12-16.

PULSE OXIMETRY

A **pulse oximeter** monitors the oxygen saturation of the blood (Fig. 12-17). **Oxygen saturation** is the percentage of hemoglobin that is saturated with oxygen. Pulse oximetry is often used during interventional procedures when sedative drugs are used because they can cause respiratory depression. A noninvasive light sensor is attached to the finger, toe, or nose to monitor the capillary blood oxygen saturation. Normal saturation ranges from 90% to 100%.

Patients with poor circulation or chronic obstructive pulmonary disease (COPD) may not have reliable oximetry readings. In addi-

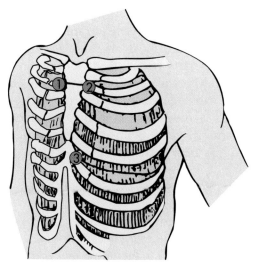

FIG. 12-16 Placement of electrodes for ECG monitoring.

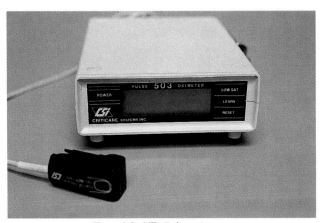

FIG. 12-17 Pulse oximeter.

tion, nail polish, bandages, increased skin pigmentation (which prohibits light transmission), and cool skin (which has decreased perfusion) are all factors that can also influence oximetry readings. The readings should be documented during procedures.

BLOOD PRESSURE

Noninvasive blood pressure measurements may be monitored with special cuffs that automatically inflate and deflate at timed intervals. Blood pressures are displayed as digital readouts on the scope.

Invasive blood pressures (blood pressures taken from within the body) may be monitored during angiographies. These measure either differences in pressure above and below narrowing in a blood vessel or a specific arterial pressure (such as pulmonary artery pressure). Invasive blood pressure measurements help reveal the presence of disease in a blood vessel. Special pressure tubing that includes a transducer is connected to the angiographic catheter. After calibration the pressure reading and waveform are transmitted to the monitor and may be recorded on graph paper.

POSTEXAMINATION ASSESSMENTS

After any procedure, patients should be evaluated again. Patients who have had biopsies should be checked for signs and symptoms of internal or external bleeding, including tachycardia, hypotension, diaphoresis (excessive perspiration), and pain. Patients who have had lung biopsies may experience hemoptysis (coughing up blood) for a short time after the biopsy. Watch them closely for excessive bleeding, pain, and shortness of breath.

After an arteriogram a patient may be in the recovery area for 30 to 60 minutes until hemostasis is achieved at the arterial site. Hemostasis can be achieved by putting hand pressure or a C-type clamp (which maintains steady pressure and permits personnel to leave the bedside) on the arteriography site. Take the patient's peripheral pulses and compare them with the pulses from the preexamination assessment.

DIAGNOSTIC MEDICAL SONOGRAPHY

Diagnostic medical sonography, or ultrasound, does not use ionizing radiation. Instead, sound waves are reflected to produce an image. Specialized equipment is needed for sonography, including **transducers,** or probes, which transmit and receive sound waves. Sound waves are transmitted into a body part. Some of the sound waves are absorbed by tissues and others are reflected back to the transducer. The sound waves reflected to the transducer are analyzed by a computer and displayed on a monitor, and the resulting images can be printed out for final interpretation (Fig. 12-18).

Diagnostic medical sonography can be used to create images of various body parts, including the abdominal and pelvic organs, the heart and blood vessels, the thyroid gland, the scrotum, the breast, and neonatal brains. It is commonly used to evaluate the fetus within the mother's uterus.

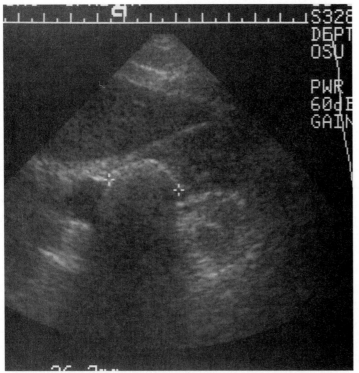

FIG. 12-18 A diagnostic medical sonogram showing stones in the gallbladder.

Although sonographic studies are usually painless, all patients must be fully informed about the specifics of the procedure (Fig. 12-19). Communicating effectively (as discussed in Chapter 2) is a vital component of a successful imaging procedure. Ultrasound produces no known side effects in the ranges in which it is used in imaging procedures. Some patients may erroneously believe that ultrasound causes high heat levels capable of burning tissue; explain to patients that this information is not true.

The success of sonographic examinations depends heavily on the sonographer's skills, and in addition, each patient is unique. Most ultrasound procedures are noninvasive and complement other imaging modalities. Sonographers must perform multiple tasks simultaneously during sonographic procedures. These tasks require intense concentration and include assessing anatomy, adjusting the sonographic instruments, and recording the pertinent images for interpretation.

TRANSDUCER CONSIDERATIONS

Different types of transducers are used to obtain images of different body parts. With experience and education, sonographers learn which transducers are appropriate for different procedures. The selection depends on the body part and the patient's body habitus. In general, high-frequency transducers are used for small body parts and hyposthenic patients. Low-frequency transducers are used for larger parts located more deeply in the body and hypersthenic patients.

Each transducer contains a piezoelectric crystal that is necessary for transmitting and receiving sound waves. Because the crystal is fragile, transducers must be handled carefully. If a transducer is dropped, the crystal or housing may break and result in costly repairs or replacement.

Transducers and probes must be cleaned between each use; take universal precautions and use aseptic technique. Clean transducers with alcohol, ethylene oxide, or betadine, but never expose them to heat. Heat sterilization affects the molecular composition of the crystal.

During procedures, always consider the patient's privacy, especially when using transvaginal or transrectal probes. These probes, which are inserted into the vagina or rectum, can provide invaluable

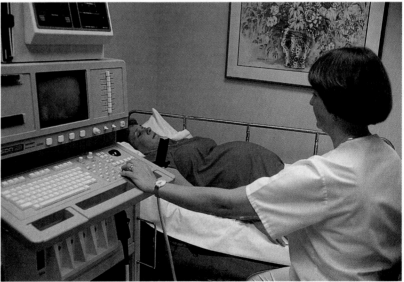

FIG. 12-19 Patients must be well informed about their ultrasound procedures before examinations begin.

information. Like all procedures, transvaginal and transrectal sonographic procedures should be clearly explained to each patient before the procedure begins. Condoms or similar protective covers should be placed over transvaginal and transrectal probes and changed for each patient. These probes must also be chemically disinfected between each use.

USE OF SONOGRAPHIC IMAGING IN INVASIVE PROCEDURES

Ultrasound is also used to localize cystic or fluid-filled areas during biopsy or aspiration procedures. Sonographic guidance is commonly used for aspirations of breast and kidney cysts and performing amniocentesis. Most biopsies and aspirations carry infection and bleeding risks. Observe patients carefully after ultrasound-guided invasive procedures for signs and symptoms of bleeding or sepsis.

MAGNETIC RESONANCE IMAGING

Magnetic resonance imaging does not use ionizing radiation; instead, instruments using magnetic fields and radio waves produce the images. Powerful, super-conductive magnets and specialized devices called *coils* transmit the radiofrequency waves and receive nuclear magnetic resonance (NMR) waves.

The patient is placed within a large magnet (Fig. 12-20); radio waves are transmitted to a particular body part. The radio waves alter the magnetic field and are absorbed by the body part. The tissues within the body resonate with the frequency of the pulsed radio wave. The resulting NMR waves are received by the coil and analyzed by a computer that displays the image on a monitor. The images may be printed out as hard copy for final interpretation (Fig. 12-21).

MRI examinations can be used to create images of various body parts, such as the abdominal and pelvic organs, heart and blood vessels, musculoskeletal system, and central nervous system. Because magnetic resonance (MR) examinations do not create images including bone, they are excellent modalities for creating images of portions of the brain and spinal cord—areas that are often hidden by the cerebral cranium and vertebral column in conventional and CT images.

Most of the patient care information described applies to MRI examinations. However, there are additional considerations for patients and technologists in MRI areas. Although MR studies are generally quite painless, each patient must be well informed about

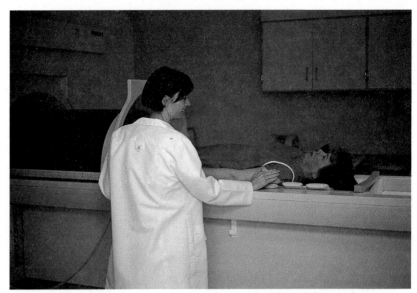

FIG. 12-20   Patient is placed in a large magnet for an MR procedure.

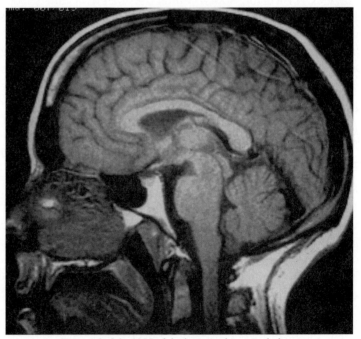

FIG. 12-21   MRI of the brain in the sagittal plane.

their specific procedure. Carefully screen each patient, all medical staff, and any visitors before entering a magnet room.

MAGNET SAFETY

All patients, visitors, and staff must be screened for contraindications to magnetic fields before each examination. Patient histories and screenings must be documented and kept as part of the patient's permanent medical record (Fig. 12-22). If a patient is unable to complete the form accurately because of physical or mental impairments, a family member, the patient's private physician, or the patient's medical records must be consulted to complete the screening process. If there are any doubts or unknowns in the patient's history, the scan should not be performed.

Make sure the patient dresses appropriately for the procedure and removes all loose metal. Secure valuables in a locker.

THE MAGNET ROOM

Magnetic-field warning signs should be posted outside all areas and rooms that contain magnetic fields greater than 5 gauss (G) indicating the hazards of high magnetic fields. Access should be limited to trained personnel, patients, and visitors who have been properly screened. No ferromagnetic equipment, tools, or objects can be brought into the magnet room. Screen objects with a hand-held magnet before they are taken into the magnet room.

Magnetic imaging devices with superconductive magnets require **cryogens** to supercool their magnets. The cryogens most commonly used are liquid helium and nitrogen. Cryogenic gases may only be handled by trained personnel. The gases must be vented outside to prevent leaking or evaporation into the magnet room. All magnet rooms must be monitored for acceptable oxygen levels and should be equipped with audible alarms that sound when oxygen levels are unacceptable. If the alarm sounds, the patient and all personnel must evacuate the room immediately, and service personnel must be notified. All trained personnel should have annual magnet safety retraining.

CONTRAINDICATIONS TO MAGNETIC RESONANCE EXAMINATIONS

Patients with known or suspected contraindications to MRI examinations or incomplete histories should not be scanned. A list of known contraindications should be available at each operator con-

The Ohio State University Hospitals Magnetic Resonance Facility
Patient History and Screening Form

NAME: _____ DATE: _____

AGE: _____ WEIGHT: _____   SEX: ____ Male ____ Female

PLEASE CIRCLE THE CORRECT RESPONSE TO EACH QUESTION:

1. Yes   No   Have you ever had surgery? What type and when? _____

    _____

    Specifically: Have you ever had surgery on the following?

Yes	No	**Eyes**	Yes	No	**Spine**
Yes	No	**Heart/Chest**	Yes	No	**Ears**
Yes	No	**Brain**			

2. Yes   No   Do you have any **metal implants** or **prostheses** inside your body?

    What type and where? _____

    Specifically: Do you have any of these implants?

Yes	No	**Cardiac Pacemaker**
Yes	No	**Brain Aneurysm Clips**
Yes	No	**Blood Clot Filter**
Yes	No	**Eye or Lens Implant**
Yes	No	**Heart Valve**
Yes	No	**Inner Ear Implant**
Yes	No	**Swan-Ganz Catheter**

_____ Magnet Implants	_____ Penile Prosthesis	_____ Insulin Pump
_____ Artificial Limb	_____ Ventricular Shunt	_____ Infusion Pump
_____ Neurostimulator	_____ Metal Clips	_____ Spinal Rods
_____ Wire Sutures or Staples	_____ Tattooed Eyeliner	_____ Wig/Hairpiece
_____ Metal Rods, Plates, Pins, Screws, or Nails		

3. Yes   No   Do you work with metal as a hobby or profession?

    Yes   No   Do you routinely wear safety goggles?

4. Yes   No   Could you have any **metal foreign objects** in your **eyes?**

5. Yes   No   Do you have any **metal foreign objects** anywhere in your body?

    Specifically: Do you have:

Yes	No	Shrapnel
Yes	No	Bullets

(continued on back)

6. Yes   No   Could you be pregnant?

                       Date of last menstrual period: _____

7. Yes   No   Are you breastfeeding?

8. Yes   No   Are you **allergic** to any drugs? _____

9. Yes   No   Why do you need an MRI? _____

You must remove all jewelry and metal items from your body and clothing prior to your exam. Please lock your personal items and valuables in the lockers and bring the key with you into the magnet/exam room. You may remove your shoes, glasses, dentures, or wig in the magnet/exam room.

One of the MR technologists will explain the MR exam to you fully and review this form with you. Please do not hesitate to ask questions.

I attest that the above information is correct to the best of my knowledge. I have read and understood the entire contents of this form and I have the opportunity to ask questions regarding the information on this form.

Signature of person filling out this form: _____

Relationship to the patient: _____

** Do Not Write Below This Line **

Reviewing technologist signature: _____

Information source: Patient   Chart   Other: _____

Attending radiologist approval: _____

FIG. 12-22 Patient history and screening form for MRI.

MAGNETIC RESONANCE IMAGING CONTRAINDICATIONS

PATIENTS WITH THE FOLLOWING DEVICES SHOULD NOT UNDERGO MRI EXAMINATIONS:

- Intracranial ferromagnetic aneurysm clips
- Pacemakers
- Pre-6000 series Star-Edwards heart valves
- Swan-Ganz catheters
- Intraocular or intracranial foreign bodies
- Insulin pumps
- Heart or Holter monitors
- Infusion pumps
- Hearing aids (must be removed)
- Bullets and shrapnel
- Tissue expanders with magnetic ports
- Biostimulators
- Lens implants with metal rings
- Cochlear implants
- Ferromagnetic IVC filters and many intravascular coils, stents, and filters
- Poppen-Blaylock carotid artery vascular clamps
- Fatio eyelid springs
- Martensitic retinal tacks

sole (box). Listings of safe and unsafe medical devices are updated regularly. You must have current information when screening patients for MR procedures.

NUCLEAR MEDICINE

Nuclear medicine is a diagnostic and therapeutic modality that uses radioisotopes or radiopharmaceuticals to create images of or treat various body systems. Nuclear medicine began in the 1950s with the discovery of technetium-99m and the development of specialized imaging devices such as the rectilinear scanner and the **scintillation camera.** Technetium-99m is the most commonly used radioisotope in modern nuclear medicine departments. Unlike conventional radiographic equipment, nuclear medicine imaging equipment (Fig. 12-23) does not create ionizing radiation; instead it detects the radioactivity emitted from the body after a radiopharmaceutical injection. The scintillation cameras work in conjunction with specialized computers designed to produce images that pro-

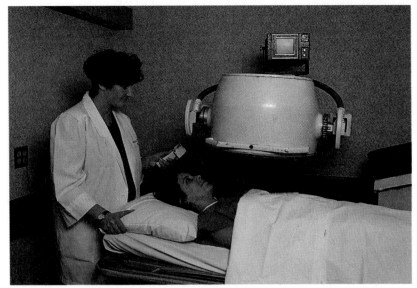

FIG. 12-23 Patient is placed under a scintillation camera for the nuclear medicine procedure.

vide information about the physiologic functioning of a specific organ or body system.

Except for the radiopharmaceutical injection, nuclear medicine studies are painless. Patients must be well informed about their specific procedure. Many patients fear radioactivity and need reassurance that the benefits from nuclear medicine studies far outweigh any risk associated with radiation exposure.

RADIOPHARMACEUTICALS

Although technetium-99m is the most commonly used radioisotope in nuclear medicine, other elements such as iodine-131 are also used. **Radioisotopes** and **radiopharmaceuticals** are specialized medications that contain radioactive elements combined with other physiologic compounds such as diethylenetriamine pentaacetic acid (DTPA), sulfur colloid, phosphates, and pyrophosphates. Because these physiologic compounds are not disturbed when combined with radioisotopes, they can travel to the body system being examined. As the radioisotope undergoes radioactive decay, it emits radiation that is detected by the scintillation camera. The radioisotope becomes a localization label for the physiologic compound of interest, allowing evaluation of the specific organ or system. Radiopharmaceuticals may be administered intravenously, orally, or by inhalation, depending on the area being examined.

Nuclear medicine studies may be performed to evaluate the thyroid gland, brain, respiratory system, liver, spleen, gallbladder, kidneys, skeletal system, and heart. Unlike conventional radiography, which primarily provides anatomic information, nuclear medicine studies provide information regarding the physiologic functioning of organs and body systems.

Technologic advances in imaging equipment and computers have led to the development of the specialized equipment found in modern nuclear medicine departments. Dual- and triple-head scintillation cameras allow multiple–body plane images to be obtained simultaneously. In single-photon–emission computed tomography (SPECT), the nuclear medicine camera rotates around patients to produce tomographic images. Positron-emission tomography (PET) provides valuable information regarding the physiologic functioning of organ systems in a cross-sectional format similar to the format of CT and MRI.

SUMMARY

The radiologic sciences offer a wide range of practice opportunities in health care settings. Whether you choose to subspecialize in a particular modality such as mammography or expand your horizons and include additional modalities such as diagnostic medical sonography or nuclear medicine, basic patient care techniques are vital. Treat each patient with respect and dignity. Communicate with patients clearly and articulately, and thoroughly explain each imaging procedure. Patients must be treated in safe, clean, and friendly environments. Imaging professionals must demonstrate compassion, competence, and concern for patients, guests, and other members of the health care team.

STUDY QUESTIONS

1. Why is communication important when performing a mammographic examination? What makes mammography patients unique?
2. Explain the importance of obtaining a thorough health history when performing a mammographic examination. Specify the major areas that must be covered.
3. Briefly explain how a CT image is produced.
4. List the advantages of CT imaging over the use of conventional radiographic imaging for medical diagnosis.
5. What types of contrast material are used in CT?
6. List three items that should be included in a preexamination assessment for angiography.
7. Describe the Seldinger technique.
8. What are the most common risks associated with invasive procedures?
9. Interventional procedures involving the biliary or urinary system carry a high risk of infection. Why?
10. An ECG shows which of the following: (a) the electrical functioning of the heart or (b) the mechanical function of the heart?
11. Describe the characteristics of a PVC.
12. Name and describe two life-threatening dysrhythmias.
13. If a flat-line waveform appears on a scope instead of a normal ECG waveform, which two things should be checked?
14. For what reason is pulse oximetry used during interventional procedures?
15. List several symptoms that may indicate a patient is bleeding internally after a procedure.
16. Briefly explain how a sonographic image is produced.
17. List three areas of the body that can be examined with images from ultrasound.
18. Describe the proper methods for handling and cleaning sonographic transducers.
19. Briefly explain the way a magnetic resonance image is produced.
20. List three areas of the body that can be examined with images from MR scans.
21. Name four contraindications to performing MR examinations.
22. List two differences between nuclear medicine studies and conventional radiographic examinations.
23. Specify five organs or body systems commonly imaged by nuclear medicine procedures.

Index